Perfect Health for Busy People

A Maharishi Ayurveda Guide to Enjoying a Longer and Happier Life

Laurina Buro Carroll

**Ayurveda Wellness Consultant
Transcendental Meditation
Teacher**

Perfect Health for Busy People

A Maharishi Ayurveda Guide to Enjoying a Longer and Happier Life

Perfect Health Press

630-903-0525

Web: https://yourayurvedaconsultant.com

Please note:

Perfect Health for Busy People is an educational service that provides general information and discussions about health and related subjects. The information and other content provided in this book, or in any linked materials, are not intended and should not be construed as medical advice, nor is the information a substitute for professional medical expertise or treatment.

Any statements made in this book have not been evaluated by the FDA, and any information or products discussed are not intended to diagnose, cure, treat, or prevent any disease or illness.

Please consult a healthcare practitioner before making changes to your diet or taking supplements that may interfere with medications.

Transcendental Meditation™ and TM™ are protected trademarks licensed to Maharishi Foundation USA, a non-profit educational organization.

Photographer: Kristie Schram

Cover Designer: George Foster

Editor and Typesetting: John Kremer

Editorial Advice: Christine Schrum

Editorial Advice: Lisa Thaler

Dedication

This book is dedicated to Maharishi Mahesh Yogi, for bringing the profound gift of Vedic knowledge to the world.

Acknowledgements

To my parents, Trudy and Nat, for sharing their ability of bringing tremendous love and laughter into our home. As the saying goes, "Laughter is the best medicine," and without any negative side effects!

To my stepparents, Linda and Tony, for adding even more love and spice to our family.

To my daughter, Olivia, whose sweetness and unconditional love have created waves of bliss in my life each and every day.

To Alfred Lopez, for teaching me the TM technique and giving me my first experience of transcending, and for helping me raise our beautiful daughter.

To my husband, Bolton, for making each and every day together so utterly joyful and fun. Your love and support mean the world to me. I'm blessed beyond words to have you in my life.

To my siblings, Pat, Paul, and Mark, for your love and excellent comedic abilities that get me through life's difficult times. You're my constant source of inspiration.

To Christine Schrum, for her excellent editorial suggestions and great insights.

To John Kremer, for his editorial suggestions and wisdom on creating an easy-to-read book. Sorry I kept you up so late!!

To my assistants, Beata, Wendi, and Simona. I can't survive without any of you. You are so devoted to my cause and each and every day you put forth your best to help me. It's greatly appreciated.

To my photographer, Kristie Schram. We had so much fun shooting. I'm in awe of your talents.

To George Foster, book cover designer, thank you for your patience with all the changes and for your expertise in creating a wonderful cover.

To all the meditators in the Chicago area, Germany, and around the world who I have trained! I feel blessed to have had the privilege to teach you this profound technique. Thank you for your trust in me. Also, to my Ayurveda students for being open to this knowledge.

To all the Vaidyas and Vedic experts trained in Maharishi Ayurveda, for their knowledge and insights.

To my mentors and colleagues at the Raj Health Spa in Fairfield, Iowa, with special thanks to Mark and Helen Toomey, Paul Morehead, Vaidya Manohar Palakurthi, and Dr. Nancy Lonsdorf.

To my mentors and colleagues at the Maharishi Ayurveda Spa in Schledehausen, Germany.

To my fellow TM teachers for your support and love.

To the beautiful ladies at the Global Mother Divine Organization.

To the David Lynch Foundation.

To Maharishi International University (MIU) for an outstanding and unforgettable university experience.

To Maharishi Foundation for giving me the opportunity to teach thousands of people the TM technique.

Contents

A Note to Readers

I'm writing this book as an experienced Ayurvedic wellness consultant and mother who has seen tremendous benefits from Ayurveda in my clients and family alike. Please note, however, that the information in this book is intended for informational purposes and should not be used as a substitute for the advice and care of a physician.

Before making any changes to your diet or exercise routine, it is wise to check in with your personal physician to ensure the suggestions are appropriate for your unique constitution. Nutritional and lifestyle needs vary from person to person. This book is not meant to take the place of a medical consultation and should not be used to diagnose, treat, or cure any disease.

Throughout the book, I share various anecdotes about my clients and their experiences with Ayurveda. For privacy reasons, all names and identifying characteristics of my clients have been changed.

Preface

Leaving the *Mad Men* Lifestyle Behind and Finding Balance Through Ayurveda

Growing up in the 1960s and 1970s, my family lived like most Americans at the time—not very health-conscious. We ate everything, good and bad. My Irish-English mother served us plenty of salads and vegetables, but there was also an abundance of red meat in the traditional Irish dishes she cooked, like leg of lamb or corned beef and cabbage. Thanks to my father—a full-blooded Italian—our plates were also piled high with pasta, bread, and sweets. We used to dip the Italian bread into the sauce while waiting for dinner, which was unbelievably delicious but tended to stick to my hips.

Processed food was growing in popularity in the U.S. at the time, and there were carbs galore in my household, including sugary foods like donuts, cookies, Twinkies, and other calorie-laden treats. Many of my family members smoked cigarettes and drank alcohol whenever there was a party or when relatives were visiting. It was like *Mad Men*—my dad drank and smoked at his lunch meetings, thinking nothing of it. Luckily, none of us ended up becoming addicted to alcohol, but looking back I was certainly hooked on sugar.

By the time I turned sixteen, I was drinking at parties and in bars; I looked older and found it easy to get into bars. I became very fond of alcohol way too young and also smoked cigarettes on and off for a few years. Eighteen was the legal drinking age back then, and most parents didn't curtail their kids' drinking or smoking since it was an accepted part of the social scene everywhere.

Looking back, I remember feeling not that great most of the time—but I didn't know what was causing it. I'd wake up groggy and a little sick after drinking with friends or eating rich, heavy foods. I worked side jobs and didn't generally drink in excess on work nights, but even small amounts of alcohol didn't agree with me. The next day, I would stuff myself with fast food for quick fuel. If I was lucky, there were some sweets around the office to nibble on when my energy plummeted mid-afternoon. I learned early on that you can get through the day high on caffeine and sugar, though it's certainly not a great long-term solution.

At nineteen, I started jogging and doing Jane Fonda workouts. The upside was that I had to quit smoking to keep up. I also cut back on my drinking. Still, it seemed like my mom and I were always being sucked into one crazy fad diet or another in an attempt to lose weight.

Technically, I wasn't overweight, but I certainly wasn't a stick-thin type like some of my slenderer friends. The Twiggy look was popular then, thanks to the ultra-slender British cultural icon and model of the same name. That didn't help the self-esteem of any young girl who, like me, had a fuller figure and a strong, athletic physique (I only came to embrace these later in life).

At the time, vitamins and supplements were becoming popular, and by the 1980s, North American society as a whole was leaning toward fitness, aerobics, and the relentless pursuit of better health. Unfortunately, extreme dieting was part of that health craze. Mom and I tried everything from the grapefruit diet to the Atkins diet and Carnation's Slender, but none of those stringent approaches really offered a balanced, healthy, and sustainable approach to eating. My quest for a healthier lifestyle continued.

At twenty-two, I finally found what I was looking for when I learned to meditate and soon thereafter discovered Ayurveda. Used successfully in India for millennia, Ayurveda employs diet, lifestyle, and herbal recommendations to strengthen the body and mind while maintaining balance. The oldest system of natural healthcare in the world, Ayurveda considers that each one of us is an individual. There's no one-size-fits-all approach to wellness (which is why fad diets are so often ineffective). Ayurveda transformed my life and made me a much healthier, happier person.

As an introduction to each of the chapters that follows, I will share my experiences with Ayurveda. I hope this sharing will help you understand how Ayurveda changed my life—and can change your life.

Introduction

Let's Get Started

Perfect Health for Busy People is exactly what it sounds like: an easy-to-use guide for living a healthy, balanced life the Ayurveda way, no matter how hectic your schedule. As someone who balanced a full-time career with the demands of being a single mother for more than a decade, I understand busy! But I think you'll find that following a few basic Ayurvedic recommendations actually helps you to feel better physically, think clearer, and enjoy more energy and emotional balance throughout the day.

My goal in writing this book was to take the ancient wisdom of Ayurveda and distill it into bite-sized bits of information you can use to improve your life *right now*—starting with this introduction. We'll begin with an overview of Ayurveda and its basic principles. Then we'll move into an understanding of the *doshas*—the elemental energies that govern the functioning of your body, mind, and emotions, according to Ayurveda.

Later in this introduction, you'll take a quiz that will help you determine your individual Ayurvedic constitution and what foods and lifestyle choices are best suited for your constitution. Later, in Appendix I, we'll go into easy and tasty Ayurvedic recipes you can whip up in thirty minutes or less to fuel yourself and your family with fresh, balancing food.

This is *your* Ayurvedic journey, and you can use this book however you like. To start cooking healthy, balancing meals tonight, flip to the recipes in Appendix I. To discover your Ayurvedic constitution right now and get some basic recommendations, go to *What's My Dosha?* later in this introduction and take the quiz.

Read the rest of this introduction as soon as possible so you're equipped with an understanding of the foundations and principles of Ayurveda, from which everything else in this book unfolds.

While *Perfect Health for Busy People* is geared toward beginners, I believe it offers something for those familiar with Ayurveda as well. In addition to covering Ayurvedic basics, we'll explore how this ancient practice can be used for modern health issues caused by genetically modified foods (GMOs) and pesticides. We will also discover why other health issues caused by parasites, viruses, and bad bacteria are more prevalent today and thus affecting our health now more than they were a few decades ago.

Ayurveda has helped me, my family, and my many wellness clients live healthier, happier, longer, and more balanced lives. The door is open. Let's enter this world of health and wholeness together.

Modern Medicine and Ayurveda

In recent years, physicians and researchers have grown increasingly curious about Ayurveda and its benefits. Promising preliminary studies have indicated that curcumin—an extract found in turmeric, a root long used in Ayurveda—may control osteoarthritis pain as effectively as ibuprofen.

A 2017 review published in the *Journal of Alternative and Complementary Medicine* found that triphala, another Ayurvedic botanical, appears to have laxative properties, supports digestion by assisting the body in absorbing nutrients, and acts as a powerful antioxidant.

Along with conventional treatments for allergies and sinus problems, the Mayo Clinic includes on its website information about *neti pots*— small, teapot-shaped devices used for saline nasal irrigation by Ayurvedic practitioners for thousands of years, as well as herbal nose oils called *Nasya* for purifying toxins from the sinus cavity and keeping them moist.

Modern research on Maharishi Ayurveda modalities is presented throughout this book including the Transcendental Meditation technique, diet, detoxification therapies, herbal preparations, and more.

As part of my work as an Ayurvedic Wellness Consultant, I meet with physicians who are interested in learning more about Ayurveda and the broader world of Complementary and Alternative Medicine (CAM). A Chicago-based medical doctor who practices integrative medicine regularly sends patients to me for consultations on healthy eating and Ayurveda.

I also give introductory presentations to physicians, hospitals, and clinics in the Chicago area. In these talks, I make it clear that I have a deep respect for the vocations of doctors and the lifesaving measures modern medicine has to offer. Often, I'll joke with them and say with all sincerity, "If something happens to me during this lecture and I lose consciousness, please hook me up to every drug and machine possible to keep me alive."

While Ayurveda is a natural system of medicine, some of the ancient texts do recommend the use of pharmaceuticals and surgery in certain situations. But, generally, Ayurveda recommends a preventative approach using meditation, diet, lifestyle, and botanicals rather than over the counter or prescription medicine. While pharmaceuticals have value, they can also create problems of their own—namely, side effects and resistance.

These days, there's a quick pill for everything: heartburn, headache, joint pain, motion sickness—the list goes on. But with every over-the-counter medicine comes a long list of unpleasant (and, when used in excess or over long periods of time, harmful) side effects. Prescription medication is no different.

Antibiotic resistance has become a worldwide epidemic. As of 2018, the World Health Organization lists antibiotic resistance as "one of the biggest threats to global health, food security, and development today." There's no disputing the fact that antibiotics *do* have an invaluable place in treating acute bacterial infections; the problem is that they're being prescribed in excess, and we're overusing them. As a result, dangerous bacteria are becoming resistant to these medications, making infections more difficult (and expensive) to treat.

In India, traditional Ayurveda households have known for thousands of years that the key to good health is simply to eat well, follow a healthy routine, stay rested and, above all, foster healthy digestion. When minor imbalances arise, they are often addressed through rest, routine, a healthy diet, and herbal preparations.

Ayurveda holds that the body has its own inner intelligence, and with a bit of support, it can usually return to a state of balance. That being said, in the case of medical emergencies and chronic conditions, seek and follow a physician's advice. These days, many physicians are open to integrative approaches that support the best of Eastern and Western medicine.

In our modern world, we have a wealth of wellness information at our fingertips: namely, the internet. That comes with pros and cons. Every week, it seems, there's some new doctor or health guru online touting their revolutionary way to shed pounds, amp up energy levels, and boost brainpower. The fad diets haven't stopped, either; if anything, there are more of them now. But, as in the 1980s, the benefits you gain from some of these regimens may only last a short period of time—or worse, actually prove harmful over the long-term.

Amidst the whirlwind of conflicting information online, Ayurveda is grounded in tradition and backed by thousands of years of successful use. Prevention is a fundamental tenet of Ayurveda and one of my chief goals as a wellness consultant. Rather than simply treating imbalances as they arise, my goal is to help you *prevent* those imbalances from arising in the first place.

A Brief History of Ayurveda

Ayurveda is the world's oldest system of natural medicine. There are signs of the cultivation of foods and spices recommended by Ayurveda during the Bronze Age in the Indus Valley between 3300 and 1300 BCE. But the Ayurveda system became formalized in writing around 400 BCE.

It is said that Ayurveda was cognized several millennia ago in India by a group of *rishis* (enlightened sages) who sought to bring good health to people everywhere. After a period of deep meditation, these holy men cognized the ancient Ayurvedic texts: the *Charak Samhita* and *Sushruta Samhita*—both said to have been written around 400 to 200 BCE.

In Sanskrit, the language of ancient India, the word *ayu* means "life" and *veda* means "knowledge." Therefore, *Ayurveda* is the "knowledge of life." In a practical sense, that means that Ayurveda offers helpful guidelines for living life in a balanced, healthful way.

Ayurveda holds that the key to a healthier, happier life lies in finding balance—not just in the body, but in the mind, emotions, and spirit as well. Sound like a lofty goal? Don't worry. With just a bit of attention to diet and lifestyle, you can move closer to balance.

Basic Principles of Ayurveda

While learning about a vast, ancient system of natural healthcare might seem like a daunting task, the basic principles of Ayurveda are actually quite simple. Below are four of Ayurveda's founding tenets, which we'll explore in depth throughout this book.

An Ounce of Prevention Worth a Pound of Cure

Benjamin Franklin actually said that, but it's the prevailing wisdom held by Ayurvedic *vaidyas* (experts) and has been since ancient times. The aim of Ayurveda is to address imbalances as they arise and prevent them from developing into chronic conditions. In essence, avert the danger that has not yet come.

Food Is Medicine

An Ayurvedic proverb states it quite well, "With improper food, medicine is of no use; with proper food, medicine is of no need." All too often, we reach for prescription medicines and over-the-counter pills when a few easy changes in diet could prevent discomfort from arising in the first place.

The Mind and Body Are Intimately Connected

These days, the mind-body connection is well recognized by scientists, but Ayurveda has known it for millennia. The mind and body have a synergistic connection and work together. Whatever your mind experiences has an impact on your body, and vice versa—which is why it's important to find balance within both.

Like Increases Like, Opposites Balance

This is a remarkably simple concept and another of the bedrock tenets of Ayurveda. For instance, when the weather is hot, we naturally crave cooling things like watermelon and smoothies, and we eat lighter fare.

It's natural and balancing. However, sometimes we might go overboard and indulge in ice cream, milkshakes, or icy beverages, which can dampen the flames of our digestive fire (*agni*), leading to imbalances. Ayurveda can help you balance your body's natural cravings and desires in a healthy way.

Prakriti: Your Ayurvedic Mind-Body Type

We're all built differently. We need different things to feel and look our best. You might thrive on high-powered cardio classes, for example, while your best friend prefers yoga. Or maybe your brother can eat anything and stay slim, while your pants start feeling tight after just a few days of pizza and pastries. It might all seem baffling, but Ayurveda has an explanation: Every one of us has a unique constitution.

We are part of nature, and nature is part of us. Have you ever noticed how your body just seems to feel better during some seasons compared to others, or in specific climates? Or that your energy ebbs and flows throughout the day? Nature's rhythms and elements have a direct and measurable impact on both mind and body. According to the ancient texts, every person has a unique combination of the five natural elements—earth, water, fire, space/ether, and wind/air—within them. This unique combination is your Ayurvedic constitution, or *prakriti*.

Your prakriti determines everything about you—your physical shape, your skin tone, your digestion, your mental disposition, and the way you process experiences, thoughts, and emotions. For this reason, we also refer to a person's prakriti as their *mind-body type*. Knowing your prakriti is the first step in creating a customized diet and daily routine that will help you thrive.

Prakriti vs. Vikriti

Your prakriti is determined at birth and generally stays the same throughout your life. However, as you age and go through different periods of life, your *vikriti*, or current state of imbalance, can change. In fact, your vikriti can change quite a lot from day to day, depending on factors like the weather, your diet, your stress levels, and your lifestyle.

Think of your body as a temple. Knowing your prakriti—your body's blueprint—gives you a solid understanding of your physiology's foundations, structure, and why it's built the way it is. Knowing how to assess your vikriti—your body's ongoing need for upkeep—helps you to maintain it at optimal levels and avert any unnecessary need for major (and sometimes costly) repairs.

The best way to determine your Ayurvedic constitution is to make an appointment with a *vaidya* (Ayurveda expert) or Ayurveda wellness consultant, who will give you a full assessment including pulse diagnosis and a thorough questionnaire. The second-best way is to take an Ayurvedic Mind-Body Quiz like the one I've included in the section on *What's My Dosha?* First, though, it's important to understand the doshas—the factors that influence your prakriti.

Pulse diagnosis is when the vaidya puts three fingers on the radial pulse located at your wrist to determine your dosha type. Subtle impulses help to determine the level of ama or toxins, which doshas are out of balance, how advanced your present health issues are, etc.

AYURVEDA

Vata

Ether — Air

Fire — Earth

Pitta — Kapha

Water

The Three Doshas: Vata, Pitta, Kapha

The *doshas* are elemental energies that govern every aspect of your physiology, from your biological functions to your mental and emotional processes. Each of the three doshas—Vata, Pitta, and Kapha—is associated with a specific combination of natural elements.

Your Ayurvedic constitution is determined by your unique combination of the three doshas. Have you ever noticed how some people seem quite literally fiery by nature? People like that tend to have a lot of Pitta dosha in their makeup. Or perhaps you have a friend who's often spaced out? That person likely has a fair amount of Vata in their constitution. Kapha types, on the other hand, tend to come across as grounded and earthy. We all have different degrees of Vata, Pitta, and Kapha within us, but most people have one clearly predominating dosha.

At this point, you now have a general understanding of prakriti, vikriti, and the doshas. Now, let's dive deeper into each dosha so you can see how each one affects your mind and body's functioning—and how to keep them in harmony.

Characteristics and Qualities of the Doshas

Vata Dosha	Pitta Dosha	Kapha Dosha
Description: Vata governs all movement in the mind and body. It controls blood flow, breathing, the elimination of wastes, and the movement of thoughts in the mind. Since Pitta and Kapha cannot move without it, Vata is considered the leader, or king, of the three doshas. For this reason, it's important to keep Vata in good balance.	**Description:** Pitta governs all heat, metabolism, and transformation in the mind and body. It controls how we digest foods, how we interpret and metabolize our sensory perceptions, and how we discriminate between right and wrong. Pitta governs the important digestive agnis—or fires—of the body.	**Description:** Kapha governs all structure and lubrication in the mind and body. It controls weight, growth, lubrication for the joints and lungs, and formation of all the seven tissues—nutritive fluids, blood, fat, muscles, bones, marrow, and reproductive tissues.

The chief site of Vata in the body is the large intestine.	The chief site of Pitta in the body is the navel region.	The chief site of Kapha in the body is the chest.
Qualities: Cool, dry, rough, brittle, light, airy, irregular, changing, moving, quick	**Qualities**: Hot, intense, penetrating, sharp, spicy, sour, oily	**Qualities**: Cold, oily, slow, moist, solid, steady, smooth
Vata Attributes: Slim, slender build, thin or brittle hair, dry and/or translucent skin, small-boned, enthusiastic, creative, talks quickly, resists routine but thrives on it, irregular sleep, vivid dreams	**Pitta Attributes**: Medium build, athletic, oily, or silky hair, ruddy complexion, prone to baldness, fiery, passionate, warm personality, sharp intellect, perfectionist tendencies, action-oriented, sound sleepers who require little rest, intense dreams	**Kapha Attributes**: Large build, big-boned, prone to gain weight and slow to lose it, smooth complexion, thick and lustrous hair, calm, easygoing, a little sluggish, grounded, steady emotions, sound sleep, tranquil dreams
Balanced Vata types are upbeat, creative dynamos with no end of brilliant ideas. They're bright, engaging conversationalists who are always on the go. Their sleep and digestion are a little delicate, but routine helps them thrive.	**Balanced Pitta types** are bright, friendly, intelligent, and accomplished. They're happy to debate any topic and eager to take on any new challenge—whether physical or intellectual. Pittas have rock-star digestion and get by on less sleep than most.	**Balanced Kapha types** are a joy to be around. Warm, loving, and soothing, they always know just what to say and when to say it. Plus, they give the best hugs. While they might lack motivation sometimes, a little spice (both literally and figuratively) does wonders.
Imbalances: Whirlwind Vata types can feel anxious, worried, overwhelmed, spaced out, and scattered. Insomnia is common among imbalanced Vata types, along with ailments like constipation, chronic pain, cardiac arrhythmias, rheumatic disorders, and diseases of the nervous system.	**Imbalances**: Fiery Pitta types can sometimes get overheated! Pittas may tend toward anger, jealousy, and short-temperedness. They may suffer from violent dreams as well as physical complaints such as stomach acidity, acne, peptic ulcers, hypertension, inflammatory bowel diseases, allergic reactions, and skin diseases.	**Imbalances**: Slow and steady Kapha types sometimes suffer from dullness, lethargy, and feeling down in the dumps. They may also experience feelings of attachment and greed. Kapha imbalances can lead to weight gain, diabetes, obesity, tumors, atherosclerosis, and diseases of the respiratory system.

What's My Dosha? Take the Quiz

As you were reading the descriptions above, you might have started to notice that you resonated strongly with one or two of the dosha mind-body types. Take the quiz below to determine your prakriti.

The best way to determine your Ayurvedic constitution, again, is to make an appointment with an Ayurvedic vaidya or wellness consultant for a comprehensive evaluation. That being said, the basic principles of Ayurveda are fairly simple. Taking this quiz will help you determine your dominant mind-body type (Vata, Pitta, or Kapha). As you go through this short quiz, circle the answer that best applies to you.

In some cases, you may feel that two answers apply. Try to stick to one answer, but give yourself half a point for answers that apply to you partially, or that are true some of the time.

Most people find they have some of all three doshas but strongly identify with one dosha type. If you find your answers are fairly evenly split between two doshas, that may mean you are bi-doshic. Some rare individuals are even tri-doshic, or evenly balanced among all three doshas.

What's My Dosha? Quiz

Build

a) I'm thin, slender, thin-boned, slim.
b) I have an average, athletic, or muscular build.
c) I have a large build, am heavy-set, and have big bones.

Hair, Complexion, and Skin

a) My skin is pale, translucent, and often dry or cool to the touch. My hair is fine and silky.
b) My complexion is ruddy, sensitive, and prone to rashes and acne. I blush and/or overheat easily. My hair is of moderate thickness (men may be prone to balding).
c) My skin is smooth, lustrous, and/or oily. I have a healthy glow. My hair is thick, wavy, and strong.

Eyes

a) My eyes are small, deep-set, or protruding, and my gaze moves quickly.
b) My eyes are medium-sized, with a sharp and penetrating gaze.
c) My eyes are large and have a soft gaze.

Speech

a) I tend to speak quickly, often jumping from one topic to another.

b) I speak in a clear, concise manner and sometimes sound a bit intense.

c) I speak in a relaxed, slow, methodical manner.

Digestion

a) My digestion is irregular, and I sometimes tend toward constipation. I often skip meals or forget to eat.

b) I have rock-star digestion and a roaring appetite. Skipping or delaying meals makes me *hangry*.

c) I love food and have a steady appetite. I sometimes overindulge in comfort eating, which results in sluggish digestion.

Joints

a) My joints are dry and tend to crackle or pop when I walk.

b) My joints are flexible.

c) My joints are healthy and well-lubricated.

Mind

a) My thinking is quick, agile, and sometimes all over the map. I'm a free spirit. I'm quick to learn, and quick to forget.

b) My mind is discerning and sometimes critical. I'm a perfectionist. I have a strong sense of right and wrong. I learn things quickly and easily.

c) My mind is steady and methodical. I'm sometimes slow to learn, but once I've mastered a skill, I'll have it for life.

Emotions

a) I'm creative and enthusiastic, but also prone to worry, anxiety, and insomnia.

b) I'm warm, friendly, and passionate, but also fiery, intense, and sometimes quick to anger.

c) I'm easygoing, mellow, and generous, but sometimes I feel dullness, apathy, lack of motivation, and down in the dumps.

Sleep

a) My sleep is irregular, and sometimes I'm prone to insomnia.

b) I fall asleep fine, but sometimes wake up in the early hours and can't get back to sleep.

c) I generally sleep soundly and peacefully.

Temperature Tolerance

a) I prefer warm, humid temperatures and climates. I feel uncomfortable in cold and chilly weather.
b) I prefer cooler temperatures and climates. I feel uncomfortable in hot and humid weather.
c) I'm generally comfortable in most temperatures, but I tend to prefer warm, dry temperatures and climates over cool and damp weather.

Results

Mostly a's: You're a Vata type.
Mostly b's: You're a Pitta type.
Mostly c's: You're a Kapha type.

While your Ayurvedic constitution generally stays the same throughout your life, your answers to some of these questions may vary somewhat depending on the season. Regardless of your dosha type, this quiz can help you determine which doshas need balancing at specific times.

Vata Mind-Body Type

Vata types are whirlwinds of dynamism and creativity, flitting here, there, and everywhere. They talk quickly and are full of bright ideas. Vata dosha is associated with the elements air and space, which makes a Vata-prominent person's mind agile, fluid, and prone to being a bit spaced out at times.

Because Vata dosha is cool, light, and dry by nature, these qualities are also prominent in the body. If you're a Vata type, you're likely slim and without much padding. When you're feeling out of balance, your hands and feet may tend to be chilly. Also, you may have a tendency toward dry skin, poor circulation, nervous tension, anxiety, hyperactivity, insomnia, and constipation.

In an office environment, Vata types tend not to stay at their desks for long (they have an aversion to sitting in one place). They love people, connection, and conversation. Vata employees can be tremendously valuable assets because they're excellent at coming up with new ideas and spurring creativity. They're often friendly, enthusiastic, and inspiring, which makes them great for reaching out to prospective clients.

Sometimes, Vata types get so carried away with their creative endeavors; they forget to eat, go to bed on time, or follow a healthy routine. Vata types can also easily get overstimulated, so it's important to make time for plenty of rest and relaxation. Following a healthy routine is one of the best things Vata-dominant people can do to stay balanced.

Tips for Balancing Vata

When it comes to balancing Vata, the three most important things are routine, routine, and routine. Breezy Vata types do well with grounding and predictability. Follow a healthy daily routine, make sure to eat three healthy meals a day (don't skip), and get to bed on time.

I have a lot of Vata in my nature. So, I like to use my Google Calendar to remind myself to meditate, exercise, eat, drink water, and get to bed on time. The rewards of following a schedule are actually helpful for all dosha types, but especially for Vatas.

One of the key tenets of Ayurveda is that like increases like and opposites balance. Therefore, to warm up Vata's chilly tendencies, favor all things cozy and comforting. Eat warm, lightly spiced, cooked foods (think soups and stews) and avoid raw or cool foods. Pass on the salads, crudités, and ice cream. Favor sweet, sour, and salty tastes, and reduce pungent (such as red radishes), bitter (many greens), and astringent (cranberries or lentils) tastes.

Cold dry weather can be uncomfortable for Vata types, so if you live in chilly climes, be sure to bundle up. Warm weather and sunny days are much more agreeable for Vatas.

Because they are prone to chilly extremities, dry skin, and poor circulation, Vata types benefit greatly from doing abhyanga (daily self-massage) with warm oil. Gentle yoga asanas (stretches and poses) and pranayama (breathing exercises) are also helpful for keeping Vata types calm, limber, and refreshed.

Pitta Mind-Body Type

Pitta types are fiery, charming, passionate dynamos who tend toward perfectionism. They have sharp, penetrating intellects, and they tackle new challenges with aplomb. Pitta dosha is associated with the element of fire, which can lead Pitta types to be hot-blooded at times.

Because Pitta dosha is hot, sharp, oily, and intense by nature, these qualities are also present in the body. If you're a Pitta type, you likely have a medium, athletic build with intense eyes, a rosy glow, and perhaps a tendency toward oily or sensitive skin. Pitta-predominant people tend to be so driven they can sometimes push too hard and overheat. Telltale signs of imbalanced Pitta include skin eruptions and rashes, acid stomach, diarrhea, and feelings of crankiness, irritability, critical-mindedness, and anger.

In the office, Pitta employees tend to be quick learners and high achievers with laser focus. Highly intelligent and articulate, they make great speakers and leaders when in balance. They have excellent organizing power and can be very charismatic. Where Vata types can't sit still for long periods of time, Pittas can stay glued to their seats when they're deeply engaged with a project or task (but just like the rest of us, they can burn out if they don't take breaks).

You've heard the expression *workaholic*? That's a Pitta tendency. Most Pittas derive extreme pleasure from their work, which is a good thing, but it can cause health problems if they overdo it and skip meals or sleep. Pittas are your typical type A personalities who want everything done yesterday. As a result, they're sometimes impatient with spacey Vata types and sluggish Kaphas.

My Pitta-dominant clients are often remarkably successful people who struggle a bit with work-life-rest balance. For this reason, many of them come to see me with classic symptoms of Pitta imbalance, like intense emotions, headaches, acid reflux, and stomach acidity (which, if left unchecked, can lead to ulcers). Everything in moderation is the key to restoring Pitta types to their bright and friendly selves.

Tips for Balancing Pitta

To keep Pitta's fiery energy from overheating, it's important to stay cool and avoid overly hot temperatures, climates, and food. Try not to work too hard and be sure to include some leisure time in every day. Stop and smell the roses—literally! Sweet fragrances and tastes are balancing for Pitta types.

As with Vata types, it's helpful to follow a daily routine, making sure to eat three healthy meals a day and getting to bed on time. Follow a Pitta-pacifying diet. Favor foods that are sweet and cooling (think juicy fruits, rice, leafy greens and other vegetables, and warm cow's milk or almond milk). Avoid hot, greasy, spicy, and acidic foods (skip the hot chilis, deep-fried foods, spices, and tomatoes when possible). Sweet, juicy fruits are especially balancing for Pitta types. Never, never skip meals, lest you become hangry!

Too much heat and humidity can make Pitta types flare up with rashes and irritability, so steer clear of the hot noon-hour sun and seek shade instead. Cool weather is much more comfortable for Pitta types, as are cooling activities like swimming and spending time in nature.

Pitta types benefit greatly from doing abhyanga (daily self-massage) with cooling oils like coconut or sesame infused with cooling herbs. Cooling yoga asanas (stretches and poses) and pranayama (breathing exercises) can help Pitta types maintain an even keel.

Kapha Mind-Body Type

Everyone loves a Kapha type! They are warm, loving, kind, friendly, generous, and nurturing by nature. Kapha dosha is associated with the elements earth and water, which is why Kapha types tend to take a slow, steady, fluid approach to most things.

The qualities of Kapha are heavy, smooth, solid, and moist. In the body, these qualities tend to manifest as a larger ample frame, beautiful glowing smooth skin, and thick and shiny hair. Of all the dosha types, Kaphas tend to gain weight easily and have a difficult time shedding pounds. They're also naturally drawn to sweets, pastries, and fatty foods, which can lead to overindulging. As friends and family members go, Kaphas have the most generous hearts. They are trusting and loyal.

In the office, Kapha-dominant people are extremely easy to get along with due to their cheerful, conciliatory nature. They're excellent, empathetic listeners and are among the most reliable employees around. You can set your watch by a Kapha person. When it comes to tackling new initiatives or learning new skills, it may take a Kapha person a little longer to catch up—but once they've mastered a skill, they'll have it for life. Kaphas do benefit from structure at work; otherwise, their sluggish tendencies make it hard to overcome inertia.

Kapha types have a hard time getting going and need encouragement— or some literal spice in their life. Kapha types do well by varying their daily routine, trying new things, and eating healthily spiced foods.

Tips for Balancing Kapha

A Kapha at rest tends to stay at rest. Easygoing Kapha types benefit from a little stimulation to get their energy flowing. Movement is a big part of that. Get up and out the door for a little vigorous exercise every day (even just a little helps). To break free from the doldrums, seek variety and new experiences. Early to bed and early to rise makes Kapha's naturally harmonious nature shine.

Because Kapha types tend to gain weight easily, they do best when they avoid heavy foods and sweets. Instead, it's better to follow a Kapha-pacifying diet, favoring fresh fruits, vegetables, and legumes. While all doshas need a healthy dose of vegetables, this is particularly true for Kapha types, who are prone to slow digestion. Light, dry, and warming foods are great for Kapha (think rice cakes, gluten-free crackers, and spiced meals). It's better to avoid heavy, oily, and cold foods (pastries, French fries, and ice cream sandwiches). Favor pungent, bitter, and astringent tastes and cut back on sweet, sour, and salty flavors.

Cold, damp weather isn't a favorite of Kaphas; warm and dry is ideal. Deserts are particularly suitable climates for Kapha. Whatever the weather, get those running shoes laced up and head outside to avoid feeling in a slump or down in the dumps. If you truly can't bear the cold, get on a treadmill or just run up and down stairs. Kapha types need more vigorous exercise than other dosha types (and perhaps also an exercise buddy since they tend to be less interested in exercise).

My husband Bolton, a Kapha type, is finally doing exercise at least five times a week with me. It wasn't easy for him to get into the routine, but the great thing about Kaphas is that once they get into a habit, they will stick with it.

Kapha types can also benefit from doing abhyanga (daily self-massage) with warm massage oil containing stimulating herbs. Invigorating yoga asanas (stretches and poses) and pranayama (breathing exercises) can help fire up Kapha types so they can greet the day with enthusiasm.

The 8 Pillars of Perfect Health

Pillar One: Transcendental Meditation

The Transcendental Meditation technique is the first pillar for perfect health, because it is the most effective at improving your health—more effective than any other natural approach to health. This is a strong statement, but there are over 700 scientific research studies to back up that statement.

Chapter one covers the benefits of this powerful technique on the mind, body, and emotions. In my experience as a teacher of this technique, it's been the most life-changing program for all my students, and it's the easiest meditation technique on the planet to learn.

Pillar Two: Diet and Digestion

Chapter two covers proper digestion, the key to good health. All experiences in life—mental, physical, and emotional—contribute to your digestive health. A healthier diet will lead to improved physical health and also increase happiness and enrich your life in so many ways.

We will also explore more deeply the three doshas: Vata, Pitta, and Kapha and why they are important for optimal health and freedom from short-term and long-term health issues.

The modern-day term *microbiome* is receiving a lot of attention these days, but Ayurveda has understood for over 5,000 years the premise that gut health is the first place to look when addressing health concerns. We will dig deep into why gut health is so important and also explore ways to improve your microbiome for optimal health.

Pillar Three: Sleep

According to a CDC report published in 2016, one out of three people in the U.S. do not sleep well or long enough. They either have trouble falling asleep, staying asleep, or both. Even those sleeping many uninterrupted hours will often say they don't feel refreshed upon waking in the morning.

The first question I ask a new client is: How is your sleep? Because I know that the quality of sleep will dramatically affect how a person feels the next day. In Ayurveda, the texts say, "The day begins the night before." Even modern medicine understands the importance of a good night's sleep. I have noticed that my clients who have the worst health issues do not sleep well. This correlation of a good night's sleep with good health is too obvious to ignore. In the chapter on sleep, you will get tips on sleeping well every night and feeling your best!

Pillar Four: Movement, Yoga, and Exercise

Chapter four covers how to best maintain strength and flexibility throughout your life without having to become a professional athlete or spending hours at the gym. You will also learn the importance of doing yoga, stretching, strength training, and cardio-vascular work a few times a week. This will reduce your risk of pain and injuries as you age.

We will also discuss younger people who are not physically active and why they should be encouraged to move their bodies regularly.

Pillar Five: Living with Nature's Rhythms

Cycles and rhythms govern all aspects of life. Chapter five covers the basic concerns you may have as you go from one season to another to maintain balance. You may live in different climates throughout the year—and your mind and body need to adjust to manage these changes. Also, each stage of life—childhood, teenager, early adulthood, mid-life, and maturity—requires adjustments in your lifestyle.

Pillar Six: Maharishi Vastu Architecture

Maharishi Vastu Architecture (MVA) is a set of architectural and planning principles assembled by Maharishi Mahesh Yogi based on ancient Sanskrit texts. Maharishi Vastu Architecture is also called *Maharishi Sthapatya Veda*, fortune-creating buildings and homes, and Maharishi Vedic Architecture.

Chapter six covers MVA rules and guidelines governing the orientation and proportions of a building. It also covers other potentially negative influences that can affect the home you live in, such as electromagnetic and radio frequency fields, toxic chemicals, mold, and radon.

Pillar Seven: GMOs and Health

Chapter covers the importance of organic food, non-GMO foods, and environmental pollution that we may consume, or which might affect our bodies. Everything covered in this chapter involves important factors in promoting better health and reducing your risk of disease.

Pillar Eight: Ayurveda Detox

Why do you need to do so much detoxing? Due to environmental pollution, your ecosystem is not what it once was. You are inundated with toxins: in your food, water, soil, and air. Chapter eight reveals how to eliminate harmful toxins from your mind and body, so you can be the healthiest you've ever been.

Chapter 1: Transcendental Meditation (TM)

Why Is Transcendental Meditation Part of the Ayurveda Approach?

When I first studied Ayurveda, the first thing I learned was that the practice of the Transcendental Meditation (TM) technique is of utmost importance for optimal health. It is the first recommendation in doing Ayurveda. Changing your consciousness is at the root of all healing in Ayurveda. The TM technique targets your consciousness at the core of who you are above any other modality of healing.

The mind and body are intimately connected. Whatever you do to the mind affects the body and vice versa. When you nourish the mind at the fundamental level of your consciousness, dramatic changes happen. Just do this technique twice a day and watch your emotions become more balanced. Your life will be transformed. Twenty minutes twice a day is a small investment of time for the benefits you will receive.

What Is Transcendental Meditation?

The Transcendental Meditation technique is a simple, natural, and effortless process that is the single best thing you can do to improve your health. It provides the deepest rest possible in the shortest amount of time, allowing your body to enliven its own inner intelligence.

Practiced for fifteen to twenty minutes twice a day while sitting comfortably in a chair with the eyes closed, it's enjoyable and can be easily learned by anyone at any age. The benefits are immediate and increase over time.

I've taught over 2,000 people the technique, ranging from children as young as four to mature adults in their eighties and nineties. Here are some of the benefits reported by the people who learned TM:

- ☐ Reduced anxiety, depression, ADD, and ADHD
- ☐ Increased self-esteem
- ☐ Lowered blood pressure
- ☐ Reduced chance of hypertension, stroke, and atherosclerosis
- ☐ Relief from headaches, including migraines
- ☐ Reduced insomnia
- ☐ Decreased anger, irritability, and impatience
- ☐ Increased focus, creativity, and motivation
- ☐ Helped children and adults on the spectrum with Asperger's syndrome and autism
- ☐ Lowered cholesterol
- ☐ Reduced insulin resistance in type-2 diabetics
- ☐ Improved harmony at home and in the workplace
- ☐ Increased revenue for companies

The Transcendental Meditation technique allows your mind to settle inward, beyond thought, to experience the source of thought—a state of restful alertness where your brain becomes more coherent and your body gains deep rest.

Think of the mind as an ocean. On the surface the water may seem very rough and turbulent, but a mile deep it's calm and quiet. This is just like the mind. People complain that their minds are too active, and they desire to calm their minds so they can think more clearly.

In TM, you contact the quiet level of the mind, which is a field of tremendous energy, intelligence, and creativity. Many parallels have been drawn between this very quiet level of the mind and the Unified

Field in physics, which is itself an underlying field in physics, the source of all fields and particles in creation.

During TM, we can access this quiet level of the mind, the optimal state of healing and rejuvenation for the body. When you come out of meditation, taking care of daily tasks becomes more effortless. Time seems to expand in the pool of calm that you created during meditation.

"Perhaps [TM's] greatest benefit is that it's relatively quick to learn and easy to master. No waiting weeks or months of practice before you see results: TM cuts right to the chase, taking only days—or for some, minutes—before one feels reprieve from their painful and overwhelming thoughts." — *Forbes* magazine

---

My Experience with the TM Technique

On July 21st, 1986, I learned the Transcendental Meditation technique. I know it might seem odd that a mental technique was the first step toward the transformation of my physical health, but it was.

There is nothing dearer to my heart than my twice-daily practice of the TM technique and how it has impacted my life. From the first meditation, I reached a level of peace, calm, and bliss that continues to grow even after so many decades. It's truly the gift that keeps on giving.

Transcendental Meditation is a simple, natural, effortless technique that was introduced to the Western world in 1959 by Maharishi Mahesh Yogi, a guru from India. From the moment I learned TM, I tapped into an oasis of inner peace that brought about such positive changes in my life I have done it for twenty minutes twice a day ever since.

I remember those early days meditating in my New York City apartment. I could hear the noise of the traffic outside and the hustle and bustle of the city, but nothing could disturb the profound silence I felt deep within the core of my being. This deep calm was not brought about by anything external—it was there inside me, without reason or cause. After some time, I realized that this silence was simply and freely available deep within myself, anytime and anywhere. This beautiful, pivotal realization transformed my life.

I used to expend a lot of energy worrying, but TM restored my sense of inner peace and gave me more self-confidence, creativity, energy, and focus to do anything I put my mind to. After learning to meditate, my cravings for junk food naturally fell away. Meditation gave me such a profound experience of happiness, balance, and peace that I simply didn't want to put anything into me that would alter those beautiful changes. The more I meditated, the more blissful my emotions and my life became. I no longer felt the need to alter my state of mind after a busy day, so I decided to give up alcohol completely (I haven't imbibed in the past thirty-two years, and I've never missed it). I even stopped drinking caffeine; my after-dinner espresso was no longer of interest.

I also noticed the benefits of the TM technique for my daughter, Olivia. She learned her Word of Wisdom (this is the children's version of the TM technique) at age four and then got her adult technique at age ten, so she has been practicing TM for most of her life. While she was a teenager, I noticed that Olivia and her friends who were trained in TM were more stable and balanced. They had fewer emotional problems and anxieties related to adolescence, such as peer pressure, low self-esteem, and expectations from teachers and parents to succeed. As my daughter matured into an adult, she was much more resilient when dealing with challenges in life. It's very comforting to me, as a mother, to know she has such a powerful tool to help her manage stress in life.

I was so impressed with the transformative effect that TM had on my life, I knew I needed to explore Ayurveda, which Maharishi Mahesh Yogi had revived around the same time he introduced TM to the West.

"TM has kind of revitalized me. It's definitely had an effect on my day-to-day enthusiasm for things. It just gives you consistency more than anything, consistency and like ... maybe a fire." — Tim Burgess, rock singer, The Charlatans

---

Why Do Doctors Recommend the TM Technique?

It may seem odd for a doctor or Ayurveda practitioner to recommend the TM technique as the first line of defense for a health issue, but it's becoming more common. There are many doctors recommending it in the Chicago area alone where I offer classes on Ayurveda and where I teach the TM technique.

Doctors and other experts in the health care field understand the importance of balanced cortisol and other hormones. When they discover that TM reduces elevated cortisol, many of them learn the TM technique and offer it to their patients as a tool for improving health. The health benefits are quite compelling, with over seven hundred scientific research studies, but one of the most impressive benefits that people gain from the TM technique is quickly feeling calmer and more focused throughout the day. The deep rest you gain during meditation provides the basis for more dynamic activity and greater mental clarity. You'll start to build up a tremendous amount of energy and vitality, and you will experience better health. You'll become more effective and efficient at work and in your home life. You'll be more patient with others, and you will enjoy more fulfilling relationships.

To get a better perspective on the opinion of the medical community regarding the TM technique, here are some statements and observations from various health professionals.

First, the National Institutes of Health (NIH) have funded many studies on TM and high blood pressure in patients suffering from hypertension. These studies led to the following statement from the American Heart Association:

> The Transcendental Meditation technique is the only meditation practice that has been shown to lower blood pressure.

> Because of many negative studies or mixed results and a paucity of available trials, all other meditation techniques (including MBSR - Mindfulness) received a 'Class III, no benefit, Level of Evidence C' recommendation. Thus, other meditation techniques are not recommended in clinical practice to lower BP at this time.

Lower blood pressure through Transcendental Meditation practice is also associated with substantially reduced rates of death, heart attack and stroke.

Transcendental Meditation practice is recommended for consideration in treatment plans for all individuals with blood pressure > 120/80 mm HG.

R.D. Brook, et. al., "Beyond Medications and Diet: Alternative Approaches to Lowering Blood Pressure. A Scientific Statement from the American Heart Association", *Hypertension*, 61:00, April 2013.

On its website, the Mayo Clinic, had this observation about TM:

"Transcendental meditation is a simple, natural technique... This form of meditation allows your body to settle into a state of profound rest and relaxation and your mind to achieve a state of inner peace, without needing to use concentration or effort." — Mayo Clinic

---

Dr. Steele Belok of the Harvard Medical School describes the effect of TM on stress in this way:

"Stress-related illness is common in modern society. According to a meta-analysis of available self-help programs, the Transcendental Meditation technique is the most effective program to reduce stress and anxiety. With this information, physicians can feel comfortable in offering the TM program to patients, knowing that they are unlikely to find a more effective stress-reduction program today." — Steele Belok, M.D., Harvard Medical School faculty

---

Dr. Cesar Molina, the medical director at the South Asian Heart Center and a cardiologist at El Camino Hospital in Mountain View, California, summarizes the benefits of the TM program for heart patients:

"I recommend the TM technique to my cardiology patients without reservation. In NIH-sponsored research, the TM technique has been shown to reduce blood pressure as much as or more effectively than many conventional therapies, without side effects and with positive side benefits. The TM technique has also been shown to reduce insulin resistance and cigarette usage." — Cesar Molina, M.D.

Finally, Dr. Norman E. Rosenthal, a world-renowned psychiatrist and clinical professor of psychiatry at Georgetown University School of Medicine, observed the following:

"The TM technique is the most effective non-drug modality for reducing stress and anxiety that I have seen." — Norman Rosenthal, M.D.

TM and Scientific Research

One of the main reasons that medical professionals are more and more interested in this technique for health is that there is a large body of scientific research on the TM technique.

Hundreds of scientific research studies (https://www.tm.org/popups-responsive/research.html) have demonstrated the effectiveness of the TM technique for the prevention of disease and the promotion of optimal health. The research has been conducted at top medical schools and published in over 350 peer-reviewed scientific journals. These studies span over forty years and have been conducted in more than two hundred independent universities and research institutions throughout the world. Many of the studies are randomized and controlled, with both a test group and a control group.

No other meditation technique has shown such a strong scientific basis demonstrating positive outcomes.

TM and Fewer Hospital Admissions

What's interesting about the TM technique is that, even though it is a straightforward mental technique, it has a profound effect on the physiology. The state of restfulness created by this mental technique causes the body to experience tremendous rejuvenation and rebalancing, so major health diseases can be avoided.

One of the most interesting studies on the effect of TM on individual health is a long-term study done by Maharishi International University in collaboration with an insurance company, Blue Cross Blue Shield. Published in *Psychosomatic Medicine* in 1987, this study showed that practitioners of TM experienced fewer hospitalizations due to major illnesses when compared to people not practicing TM.

Some highlights included:

☐ 87% fewer admissions for heart disease among TM practitioners

☐ 66% fewer admissions for cancer among TM practitioners

☐ 93% fewer admissions for nervous system disorders among TM practitioners

In other words, it appears that practicing the TM technique can significantly reduce your chance of developing major diseases.

TM in a Medical School

In 2014, Loyola University Chicago Stritch School of Medicine became the first major medical school in the country to include the TM program as part of its curriculum. Dr. Linda Brubaker, then dean, decided to include the TM program after reviewing the research on the technique and learning it herself. She explained: "There's no risk to this, and we really care about our medical students, and we want our students to learn self-care so they can be resilient doctors, and Transcendental Meditation is one of the things that can help them get there."

One of the medical students who learned the technique described the benefits she noticed:

"That first day I just had such a calm and clarity and extreme rest. I think that's one of the things that's most appealing ... you have this profound rest that I think most people don't even get when they go to sleep—and you have it in 20 minutes.

"I think most of the students who have taken the course and stuck with it have found it equally as life-altering. A lot of students had migraines, and since they started TM, they don't have migraines anymore because they were triggered by stress."

Maura Tresch, another student who learned at the Stritch Medical School, explained how this could help patients: "By recommending TM, we can inoculate our patients against stress and its associated effects. With TM we do not 'manage' stress—we get rid of it. With the stress gone, the health of the body and mind can improve. This is the essence of preventive medicine." (*Chicago Tonight*, WTTW, Feb. 26, 2016).

TM and Cortisol: The Stress Hormone

Why is TM so good at removing stress?

Scientists have taught us that stress is the major culprit in practically all health issues. If we want to understand stress better, it's important to look at the hormone in the body that is correlated with stress—cortisol. Your doctor may have said that you have high or low levels of cortisol. Either too high or too low is not good. The TM technique will balance cortisol, no matter which end of the spectrum you may be on.

It's crucial to have balanced levels of cortisol for optimal health. When cortisol is at a normal level, you will have higher and more normal levels of serotonin, a neurotransmitter that regulates your mood and feeling of well-being. When cortisol is too high, doctors might prescribe anti-anxiety medications and antidepressants. These medications will successfully reduce your cortisol and also increase serotonin and other neurotransmitters, but they will often cause negative side effects.

Most of the people I teach TM to prefer not to take medications for anxiety, especially over the long term. They are seeking natural alternatives. They report that medications make them feel dull and tired. And they complain of other problems such as stomach, mood, and digestive issues.

If cortisol is high, people become stressed and report continually being in a fight-or-flight mode. They can feel depressed, moody, irritable, and impatient.

Just one twenty-minute sitting of the TM technique reduces cortisol by 30 to 40%. Seven to eight hours of sleep only reduces cortisol by 5 to 10%. That's why people may wake after a good night's sleep and still feel anxious and unrested. Almost everyone who learns TM feels calmer after one session because of a dramatic reduction of cortisol.

TM and Sleep

A key benefit of the TM technique is the improvement it brings to sleep. This improvement is completely in line with the principle that deep rest from the technique helps to rebalance your physiology and mind. Part of this rebalancing is experienced as more restful sleep.

When the TM technique was first introduced to the U.S. in the 1960s, many articles in the press indicated how great the technique was for reducing insomnia. Several scientific studies have confirmed the benefit to sleep. A study done at the University of Alberta in Canada found that the average time to fall asleep for insomnia patients dropped from 75 minutes to 15 minutes after 30 days of practicing the TM technique (*Scientific Research on TM, Collected Papers*, vol 1: 41, pp 296-298).

In my experience teaching TM classes, I have been amazed by how quickly students report improvements in their sleep. In virtually every class, several students notice that their sleep has improved, even in the first few days. One student reported that ever since she began TM, she was able to stop relying on sleep aids.

"I have terrible insomnia, and about a year ago I started doing TM. After four days of doing TM, I could suddenly sleep. It was crazy. You don't need the Ambien! You can sleep magically all of a sudden!"
— Lo Bosworth, actress

TM and the Brain

What is also unique about the TM technique is its effect on brain waves. TM produces a state of restful alertness, where the mind is extremely relaxed and yet still alert or awake. This translates into a unique style of brain wave activity.

Many scientific studies have measured the electrical activity or EEG of meditators during the practice of TM.

One study found that during the TM practice alpha waves (a slow frequency of eight to twelve cycles per second) increase in the pre-frontal cortex of the brain, the section of the brain that deals with executive function or decision-making. This finding confirms that the active mind goes into a state of greater restfulness during TM, along with a state of alertness.

Another study found an increase of brain wave coherence between different parts of the brain during the practice of TM. This change in brain waves means the electrical activity of the brain is more coordinated among the different parts of the brain, and this correlates with an increase in intelligence and mental performance.

A third study found that the brain wave coherence during the practice of TM starts to carry over into the active state of the brain after TM, when an individual has practiced the TM technique for several months. Regular practice of TM can create an increase in brain wave coherence that will last well beyond the meditation session. That will transform the functioning of the brain throughout the rest of the day into a more orderly pattern, which helps improve overall mental ability.

All of these changes in the brain happen spontaneously without any effort on the part of the practitioner to create change in their brain. Increased coherence seems to grow over time, so there is a cumulative benefit from maintaining regular TM practice over time.

TM Is for Everyone, Ages 4 to 100

TM is an amazingly simple technique to learn, which is why it can be practiced by all ages, children as young as four as well as adults in the later years of life.

TM for Children

Children ages four to nine receive a different meditation technique due to their younger nervous system. They receive a walking technique called the Word of Wisdom, which they practice silently in their minds while they are walking with their eyes open for five minutes.

At the Maharishi School (for grades K through twelve) in Fairfield, Iowa, all students practice TM as part of the school routine. Each day, they meditate together by walking in silence through the halls of the school. It's quite something to experience. Oprah Winfrey filmed the students doing this. Where else would you find school children so young being silent in the halls?

The children receive a sound, called a *mantra*, when they learn the technique. This sound is very soothing for their nervous systems. They, too, experience stress dissolving, so they become eager to continue the practice with their classmates. It's actually good to get the nervous system of children acclimated to TM at a young age, so they don't build up stress.

TM for Teenagers and College Students

For teenagers, the key benefits they receive from TM are reduced anxiety and increased mental clarity. These benefits are particularly important when dealing with school and adolescent stress.

With students, research shows that practicing TM leads to increased IQ, improved memory, increased focus, increased problem solving, increased creativity, and improved academic performance. These changes, when combined with a reduction in anxiety and an increase in self-esteem, make student life much more successful and fulfilling.

Brian, a 16-year-old sophomore in high school, learned TM to alleviate his anxiety. Achieving higher performance was not even on his mind since his anxiety was so high. He was a shy, quiet young man who loved to play golf.

At the time he learned TM, Brian was getting ready to try out for the golf team at school. He didn't choose that specific week to learn because of the tryouts; that week simply worked out as the best time for him and his dad to learn.

The first day after TM training, he reported that his anxiety was less and that he did well during golf practice. The second day after training, both his anxiety and golf game got better. The last day of class, he reported that he had played his best golf ever. Although he was a sophomore, he made the varsity team while his brother, a senior, made the junior team.

For some reason, his brother had not been available to be trained in TM that week. I felt bad about that, but happy for Brian. He was now beaming with confidence.

TM and Inner-City Schools

Another area of promise for TM practice is in the field of education, where the Quiet Time program funded by the David Lynch Foundation (founded by film director David Lynch) has taught TM to students in hundreds of low-income schools around the world. Studies consistently show improvements in academic performance for these students, along with significant reductions in anxiety and disciplinary infractions.

Visitation Valley, a middle school located in a neighborhood with one of the highest crime rates in San Francisco, started the Quiet Time program. A UC Berkeley public policy professor summarized the effect of TM in this school in an article for the *San Francisco Chronicle*: "In the first year of Quiet Time, the number of suspensions fell by 45 percent. Within four years, the suspension rate was among the lowest in the city. Daily attendance rates climbed to 98 percent, well above the citywide average. Grade point averages improved markedly."

In 2014, when the program had already been underway for many years, Visitation Valley scored higher for happiness than any other school in San Francisco, regardless of socio-economic background, on the annual California Healthy Kids Survey. WestEd, the research agency that administers the survey, reported, "A prime source of happiness at Visitation Valley is Quiet Time, a stress reduction program used at several Bay Area middle and high schools."

I had the good fortune of teaching TM in a school in Chicago for the David Lynch Foundation. I saw firsthand the transformation of students in an extremely low-income, high-crime area. Many parents thanked me for the incredibly positive changes they had seen in their children due to the program.

One day when I was struggling to get a class of seventh and eighth grade students to settle down to begin their daily practice of TM, my New York heritage came out. I told the students, "If you truly don't want to meditate any more, then we will just stop the program, so think about it and let me know," and then I walked out.

As I left the classroom, a young boy ran after me and pleaded with me not to cancel the program. He loved his meditation and he really didn't want to stop it. That reinforced how much this technique was being appreciated by these kids in school.

TM and ADHD

TM has also had a profound effect on ADHD (Attention Deficit Hyperactivity Disorder). It is not surprising that TM helps students with ADHD improve their ability to focus and learn, since TM reduces stress and improves overall brain functioning.

Research published in *Mind and Brain: The Journal of Psychiatry* in 2011 confirmed the beneficial effect of TM on ADHD. The study, done on a group of ADHD students between the ages of eleven and fourteen, found that ADHD students don't experience that it is difficult to learn TM. That's reasonable since the technique does not require concentration and is known to be easy to learn.

After three months of practice, these students showed significant improvements in brain function measures associated with hyperactive symptoms. Five specific ADHD symptoms improved: ability to focus on schoolwork, organizational abilities, ability to work independently, happiness, and quality of sleep.

One of the authors of the study, Dr. Sarina Grosswald, a cognitive learning expert, commented: "In ADHD students, we saw dramatic reductions in stress with the Transcendental Meditation technique. Teachers reported that students were more ready to learn, more focused, and more confident."

TM and Working Adults

TM is extremely helpful to people in the workplace, both on a personal level and for company success. The reduction in stress, increase in energy, and heightened mental clarity lead to improved performance at work.

Many successful business executives have learned the TM technique and have incorporated the technique into their businesses. One example is Ray Dahlio, founder of Bridgewater Associates, one of the largest hedge funds in the world. He has been touted for his successes on the cover of *Forbes* magazine. In 2017, he wrote a best-selling book called *Principles*, where he discusses his forty-year TM practice and attributes his success to the practice.

He says the TM practice allows him to settle down and makes him feel like a ninja, a highly skilled competitor. During his workday, things come at him more in slow motion, so he can process them more easily and make better decisions. As a result, Dahlio has introduced the TM program as a benefit to all employees at Bridgewater Associates.

Dahlio's overall conclusion about the benefit of the TM program is contained in this quote: "Transcendental Meditation is the single most important reason for any success I have had in my life."

Another business executive who has experienced the benefits of TM is Barry Summer, former CEO of Wealth Management at J.P. Morgan. In his own words, Summer explained why he started the practice:

"Ten years ago, I met someone who practiced TM. I saw a transformation in this person's life. What I saw professionally was incredible, but more importantly, I know this person socially, and watched the way he interacted with his children, his wife. I've known this person for 30 years. I saw a different person. When you looked at him, he was completely present, happy. He introduced me to someone who taught me how to meditate. I've been a passionate meditator, twice a day, for 10 years. I very rarely will miss an opportunity to meditate. It was transformational." — Barry Summer, speaking at *Fortune Magazine*'s Annual Brainstorm Health Conference, May 2017

Most companies that have offered the TM technique to their employees have seen firsthand the benefits. Some research studies have backed their findings: greater performance, more focus, and more creativity that has resulted in higher revenue, improved harmony among workers, and greater job satisfaction.

Oprah Winfrey discussed her experience introducing TM to her business, Harpo Studios, on the *Dr. Oz* show:

"I brought Transcendental Meditation teachers into Harpo Studios to teach me and my team how to meditate. So, we started meditating. Seven of us led to 70, led to 270, led to now everyone in the company meditates. Nine o'clock in the morning and 4:30 in the afternoon no matter what is going on, we stop, and we meditate... And you can't imagine what has happened in the company. People who used to have migraines, don't. People are sleeping better. People have better relationships. People interact with other people better. It's been fantastic." — Oprah Winfrey, *The Dr. Oz Show*, Dec. 7, 2011

TM can transform the work environment. Nancy Slomowitz, CEO of a Maryland-based business consulting firm, who encouraged half of her employees to learn the TM program, shared her experience.

"The introduction of TM has totally revolutionized the atmosphere in the company, leading to better interactions between the staff, which has been more unified as a group... They have shown greater productivity and ability to carry out their activities, while remaining focused and calm." — quoted in *Transcendence: Healing and Transformation through Transcendental Meditation* (2011), by Norman E. Rosenthal, M.D.

TM and the Elderly

Interesting research studies have been done specifically on TM and the elderly. As with the other age groups, TM can benefit older people in terms of mental abilities and physical health. It is not difficult for the elderly to learn and practice this simple technique.

A controlled study done over thirty years ago at Harvard University compared elderly individuals practicing TM with other people not practicing TM ("Transcendental Meditation, Mindfulness, and Longevity: An Experimental Study with the Elderly," *Journal of Personality and Social Psychology*, 1989).

The study concluded that older meditating individuals felt younger, had sharper mental powers, and felt better about themselves than non-meditators. In addition, when following up with the groups three years after the beginning of the study, the group practicing TM had a higher survival rate than the other group, which implies that TM might lengthen peoples' lives.

Another study found that older people practicing TM showed a faster response to visual stimuli compared to a control group which was not practicing TM. This faster response, known as shorter latency, is an indication of healthy aging (*Psychophysiology*, 1989).

TM and Athletes

People who are drawn to TM are often those seeking relief from stress and anxiety. However, the technique is also a great tool for athletes who just want to gain an extra edge in their athletic performance.

The reason TM is so helpful to athletes is that it increases mental focus, reduces mental anxiety, provides increased energy, and transforms brain wave activity into a more coherent state, which translates into a heightened level of mental performance.

Barry Zito, a professional baseball pitcher who won the Cy Young award in 2002 and helped the San Francisco Giants win the World Series in 2012, attributes much of his professional success to his practice of TM. He first learned the technique in 2011 and described it in the following way: "TM helps at a core level. It's like taking vitamins so you don't get sick... Meditation erases the stress before it can take hold. It gives me the perspective to not take angry comments by strangers personally."

In his next comment, he describes how TM helps an athlete enter into the zone while engaged in competition: "I feel like I'm in a bubble of serenity, going through my deliveries one at a time. All around me is craziness, even sixty feet away there's something I could be fearful about—but I'm staying in that bubble of solitude and calm, which comes from my practice of Transcendental Meditation." (Sirius XM radio show, *Success without Stress*, October 2014).

TM and Veterans

In recent years, the military has shown a growing interest in reviewing and incorporating the TM technique to aid the treatment of veterans suffering from *post-traumatic stress disorder* (PTSD). It is a good fit for veterans, since the technique is easy to learn, is highly effective at reducing stress, and can be practiced on their own. Here are the results of a couple of research studies on TM and veterans.

One study of a group of veterans of the Vietnam War showed a 52% reduction in anxiety symptoms, a 46% drop in depression, and a 40% reduction in symptoms of PTSD after three months of practice. Some other findings were improved sleep and reduced alcohol abuse (James S. Brooks and Thomas Scarano, "Transcendental Meditation in the Treatment of Post-Vietnam Adjustment," *Journal of Counseling & Development*, 1985).

A more recent study of veterans from the wars in Iraq and Afghanistan showed a 48% reduction in symptoms of PTSD and an 87% improvement in depression after two months of practicing TM (Joshua Z. Rosenthal, et. al., "Effects of Transcendental Meditation in Veterans of Operation Iraqi Freedom with Post-Traumatic Stress Disorder: A Pilot Study," *Military Medicine*, 2011).

In 2013, the U.S. Department of Defense funded a $2.4 million clinical trial to evaluate the TM program as a treatment for PTSD. The results from this study, presented in 2017 at a Military Health System Research Symposium, concluded that TM was the most effective program to significantly decrease trauma symptom severity and depression among veterans suffering from PTSD. The TM technique was compared to what was considered the gold standard treatment at the time, which was *prolonged exposure therapy*, where subjects were exposed to the feared object in a controlled setting. One researcher preferred TM to prolonged exposure since those veterans using TM showed a more significant improvement and were not exposed to anxiety during the treatment ("Non-trauma-focused meditation versus exposure therapy in veterans with post-traumatic stress disorder," *Lancet Psychiatry*, 2018).

Paul Downs, a Marine Corps veteran who learned the TM technique, explained its effect on his life:

"After eleven years in the Marine Corps and multiple tours overseas, I got out. And when I hung up the uniform I kind of fell apart. The traumas that I brought into the Marine Corps caught up. That led to a pretty detailed plan for suicide.

"I realized that that's not my birthright, and actually I needed to try something different. ... I was introduced to a variety of different modalities, and I'd say one of the most pivotal was Transcendental Meditation. ... Focusing on the twenty minutes twice a day of Transcendental Meditation, I now have the connection to self that I didn't have before. I know who I am. And because of that realization, I now find myself as a Warrior PATHH guide at Boulder Crest Retreat. ... TM is so pivotal. You can take it anywhere. It's literally the one you can take anywhere you go.

"I found peace with my past. I realized who I am—and there's no pill for that. It is hard to believe that 20 minutes, twice a day, is exactly what we require. But it is. It works for me, and for thousands of my brothers and sisters. It has given me the opportunity not just to survive on earth but thrive here—and to live a life that is truly full of purpose, meaning, connection, and service." — Paul Downs, in testimony before a hearing "Overcoming PTSD: Assessing VA's Efforts to Promote Wellness and Healing," U.S. House Committee on Veterans' Affairs, June 7, 2017

TM in the Prisons

Prisoners often suffer from post-traumatic stress disorder. For that reason, TM has been taught in prisons for over thirty-five years. Research studies done on prisoners using the TM technique have found many benefits.

- ☐ TM reduces *recidivism rate* (rate of returning to prison) by over 30%, with some studies showing a reduction of as much as 47%.
- ☐ TM reduces the number of rule infractions in prisons.
- ☐ TM reduces criminal thinking, psychological distress, and trauma symptoms.
- ☐ TM reduces anxiety, depression, fatigue, and anger.

☐ TM increases well-being, optimism, and purposefulness.

These studies have been published in *Criminal Justice and Behavior, Journal of Criminal Justice*, and *Journal of Offender Rehabilitation*.

In a recent program in an Oregon prison, one of the inmates described his experience with TM:

"As I entered the 24th year behind bars, I had come to grips with most of the demons of the past but still felt fragmented. Recently I was given the chance to learn TM. ... As the weeks passed, that sense of fragmentation started to flow into something deeper and new. A quiet that feels so natural and restful that I feel like I've finally come home. To a place where things make sense and I'm just happy. The pains of my life haven't gone away ... just feels like I've grown beyond them."

Introducing this program to the prison population can not only alleviate a lot of human suffering by reducing recidivism, but it can also cut the size of the prison population and the cost of housing prisoners.

TM vs. Other Meditation Practices

People often ask how TM is different from other types of meditation. My response to this question is that TM is far easier to practice as well as far more effective in reducing stress and creating coherence in brain waves. No other meditation technique is able to reduce cortisol as much as the TM technique, and no other meditation technique has as many positive scientific research studies as the TM technique.

What I have learned from students who have tried other techniques is that those techniques require more focus and more effort when compared to the effortlessness of the TM technique. Students often report being frustrated by other techniques, and they find that their anxiety is increased instead of reduced.

One type of meditation called *mindfulness* involves a constant monitoring of the mind. Some meditators who have learned mindfulness report that they enjoyed it to a degree but longed for something more. Once they learned TM, they noticed a dramatic difference in the depth of their meditations: It took them a longer time to achieve a deeper state with mindfulness than with TM. Also, most reported greater benefits outside of meditation with TM than with a mindfulness practice.

One woman had been meditating using other techniques for over twenty years. She had been to India many times, went on long spiritual retreats, and learned probably every technique on the planet on a quest for inner peace, but to no avail. She was never truly satisfied.

During her first session of TM training, I asked her how she liked the TM technique. She replied in a stern voice, "It's an absolute tragedy."

I was taken back by the answer since there was a long silent pause, and I thought I might be in for a list of complaints. Instead, she continued, "It's as if I've never meditated before. Now this is meditation. This was truly profound."

She spoke for a long time just not understanding why nothing she had ever done before took her to the depths of the mind like TM. She continues to be in awe of TM's simplicity and effectiveness. Her search was over. She finally found inner peace and began to enjoy life more.

Endorsements of the TM Program

"Meditation has been a great tool for me in my life. It helps to quiet my mind and helps me see things more clearly. It brings a sense of peace to my day.... Meditation provides me space to re-balance and re-focus when things are at their busiest.... I feel a big difference in my mood when I practice regularly. I love it! It helps us become more aware; it brings wisdom and healing.... I have been meditating since my early twenties and I must say that words do not express enough the significance of its gifts in my life." — Giselle Bundchen, producer and fashion model

---

"Through meditation on a daily basis, I get to strip away the masks that we build—that I build for myself, small and large—to reach the feeling of my true self. 'Oh, this is who I really am! This is how I can experience life!' My guiding principle has become being true to myself. I used to have lots of rules... No more." — Hugh Jackman, actor

---

"I start the day with Transcendental Meditation. It puts me in the best mood. I wake up and just prop myself up in bed for 20 minutes. It's the only time my mind gets absolute rest....It's changed my life, it's changed how I think about things. I meditate before I write a song before I perform. I feel my brain open up and I feel my most sharp. When I do it, I literally can feel the neuropathways in my mind opening up. It's almost like a halo is created around my head and things just start vibrating again." — Katy Perry, singer

"I learned TM, the Transcendental Meditation technique. And it was exactly what I needed! The thing that blew me away the most about it was that it was the easiest thing I've ever done—not the easiest meditation, but the easiest thing I have ever learned. And I learn a lot of things, you know; that's my job! TM is so simple to learn; it's so simple to practice. Yet the amount of restoration that comes to you—the benefit across your life—well, it has changed everything." — Cameron Diaz, actress

"I've been doing Transcendental Meditation for over 40 years.... Doing TM will help you to take things more easy.... Do you know how I was describing TM to somebody? It's like having... you know, your phone has a charger, right? It's like having a charger for your whole body and mind. That's what Transcendental Meditation is!" — Jerry Seinfeld, comedian and actor

How to Learn TM

The Transcendental Meditation technique is taught by certified teachers through a systematic course of personalized instruction. It includes extensive follow-up and support, ensuring that everyone who learns gains maximum benefit. For information, visit https://www.tm.org.

Chapter 2: Diet and Digestion

When my daughter, Olivia, was born in October of 1987, my husband and I wanted to give her the best chance possible at a healthy and happy life. Happiness is a big part of good health. If we are not healthy, happy, and vital, we may fall short of fulfilling our desires and dreams in life. I didn't want that for my daughter.

Fortunately, I was living in New Mexico at the time and connected with Dr. Vasant Lad—a medical doctor, Ayurvedic physician, and director of The Ayurvedic Institute in Albuquerque. He helped me learn more about how to keep my family healthy by following an Ayurvedic diet and lifestyle, and by using gentle, natural Ayurvedic herbal preparations when imbalances arose.

When Olivia got sick, I gave her the herbs Dr. Lad recommended, along with lots of rest, and she responded well. Instinctively, I wanted to avoid giving her pharmaceuticals whenever possible, knowing that antibiotics are often overprescribed, and over-the-counter medications can come with unpleasant side effects. That being said, I certainly wouldn't have hesitated to take her to the ER if she'd had a dangerously high fever or other acute symptoms; I understand and respect the lifesaving value of Western medicine.

Olivia did come down with the usual battery of mild colds, swollen tonsils, and sinus issues, but my husband and I were able to treat them naturally. We fed her a lacto-vegetarian, largely organic diet with plenty of fresh vegetables, fruits, nuts, and seeds—and watched her thrive. She rarely got sick.

Simple Ayurvedic Principles That Make a Big Difference

An ancient Ayurvedic proverb states: "When diet is wrong, medicine is of no use. When diet is correct, medicine is of no need." As an Ayurvedic wellness expert, I've seen simple dietary changes transform people's lives and health for the better, again and again. The converse is true, too. All too often in our busy lives, a healthy diet is the first thing to go.

Frank, a man in his late fifties, came to me for a wellness consultation complaining of anxiety and irritability—especially in the mornings. I offered him some simple diet and lifestyle changes, and a few days later his wife emailed and said, "My husband is a new man!"

When I asked her what she meant, she replied immediately, "He started eating breakfast, and now we don't argue in the morning anymore."

What a difference one small change can make.

For 30 years, Frank had been skipping breakfast and sometimes lunch, which really threw his blood sugar out of balance, resulting in rapid mood swings. He and his wife had battled endlessly over his mood swings each day. Making matters worse, Frank is a Vata type. More than any other dosha, Vatas thrive on routine and need regular meals to stay balanced. Now, Frank starts his day with a warm bowl of cereal with nuts and dates, which has made a vast improvement in his life—and in his wife's life, too!

Food really is medicine. But it's not just about what you eat—it's also about when you eat and how well you digest. This chapter will cover guidelines on what foods are suitable for your unique constitution, along with some easy ways to kickstart your digestion.

Good Digestion: The Key to Good Health

From the perspective of Ayurveda, good digestion is crucial to good health. A strong, robust *agni* (digestive fire) helps you to maximize the nutrients you take in through your food, sending nourishment to the seven *dhatus*, or tissues, of the body: *rasa* (plasma), *rakta* (blood), *mamsa* (muscle), *medas* (fat), *asthi* (bone), *majja* (marrow/nerve), and *shukra* (reproductive tissue). When your digestion is strong, it supports all the other systems in your body.

Some of the obvious signs of healthy digestion include clear skin, pleasant breath, good energy, and a balanced mood. But healthy digestion does more than simply help your body function optimally. It also leads to the production of a very refined substance called *ojas*—the most refined product of digestion, the key to radiant health and vitality.

"It is the ojas that keeps all living beings refreshed. There can be no life without ojas. It marks the beginning of the form of the embryo. It is the nourishing fluid of the embryo and it enters the heart right at the beginning of its initial formation. Loss of ojas amounts to the loss of life itself. It sustains life and is located in the heart. It constitutes the essence of all the dhatus. The life force prana owes its existence to it." — *Charak Samhita*

Ojas and Ama: The Dance of Two Opposites

What a beautiful expression by *Charak Samhita* to introduce ojas. Directly translated, *ojas* means "that which invigorates." The most refined product of digestion, ojas is considered vitally important in Ayurveda. Ayurvedic texts teach us that an abundance of ojas in the body leads not just to good health and clear thinking, but also vibrance, vitality, radiance, and the ability to perceive higher states of consciousness.

Babies generally have an abundance of ojas at birth. This is why we are so drawn to them with their clear eyes, their radiant glow, and their soft, smooth cheeks. They also have a natural sweetness and pleasant smell to them, which just makes us want to cuddle them all the more.

No matter a person's age, we are drawn to those with a healthy glow. This natural vibrance comes from ojas, the product of healthy digestion.

Signs of Abundant Ojas in the Body

If some of the items on this list apply to you, you likely have strong digestion and an abundance of ojas in your system.

- ☐ Radiant skin
- ☐ Youthful glow
- ☐ Clear eyes
- ☐ Clear, pink tongue in the morning
- ☐ Strong healthy digestion and regular elimination
- ☐ Waking up feeling refreshed and upbeat in the morning
- ☐ Positive outlook on life
- ☐ Natural resilience to stress
- ☐ Mental clarity
- ☐ Strong immunity

When your digestion is not tip-top, your ojas can become depleted. Poor digestion often leads to poor elimination—the first step in the path toward illness, according to Ayurveda.

Healthy, daily bowel movements rid the body of waste and prevent *ama*—a sticky toxic substance that can accumulate in the body and mind as a result of poor diet, weak digestion, or external pollutants. When there's a buildup of ama in the body, it can manifest as unpleasant physical, mental, and emotional symptoms, ultimately leading to disease. In Ayurveda, it is said that poor digestion is the root cause of all disease.

Because ama is by nature a gooey substance, it can clog the body's *srotas* (channels) if left unchecked, leading first to discomfort, then to chronic illness, and finally to serious illness. If a person has arterial blockages caused by a buildup of plaque, for instance, the condition didn't happen overnight; that accumulation of impurities was years in the making.

A buildup of ama can also be expressed in unpleasant emotions, making you feel dull and lethargic or giving rise to mental health complaints, such as anxiety or depression.

Signs of Excess Ama in the Body

Do you frequently experience some of the following symptoms? If so, you may have an accumulation of ama in your body. But fear not! Help is on the way.

- ☐ A white, sticky coating on tongue in the morning
- ☐ Waking up feeling tired and dull, even after a good sleep
- ☐ Achy joints, especially in the morning
- ☐ Weak appetite or always hungry
- ☐ Excess mucus and congestion in the respiratory system
- ☐ Rashes, acne, and other skin irritations
- ☐ Losing or gaining weight too quickly
- ☐ Food cravings or being never quite satisfied
- ☐ Digestive discomfort, whether belching, flatulence, burping, constipation, or diarrhea
- ☐ Feel tired after eating, or heavy and bloated
- ☐ Mood swings
- ☐ Insomnia

If some of the symptoms on this list sound familiar, your digestion could probably use a tune-up. Fortunately, Ayurveda offers simple, practical steps you can take to strengthen your digestion and elimination to reduce ama while increasing ojas.

Making the decision to improve your health through proper diet and digestion takes some commitment. But proper digestion can improve the quality of your life to such a vast degree that it's definitely worth it. Many of my clients tell me that they feel healthier and look younger in just a few weeks. They report that they feel better both physically and emotionally. Sound good? Let's go.

Digestion-Boosting Basics

What you eat is important in Ayurveda, and that will be covered later in this chapter. But when and how you eat also play a huge role in keeping your digestive fire robust and strong. Good digestion helps you assimilate the nutrients from your food, thus promoting ojas (vitality) and preventing ama (toxins) from accumulating in your system.

Here are the most fundamental principles of Ayurvedic eating to strengthen your digestive fire, or agni.

- ☐ **Eat three meals a day** around the same time every day. This way, your digestive fire is always primed and ready.

- ☐ **Avoid snacking and grazing.** It's better to eat a full, balanced meal and then give your body plenty of time to digest and assimilate it. If you snack throughout the day, you never give your body's systems time to reset, which weakens agni over time and can lead to an accumulation of ama. Allow three to six hours between meals to give your body adequate time to process food.

- ☐ **Chew your food well!** Wolfing your food down can lead to indigestion. Remember: digestion starts in your mouth.

- ☐ **Eat your biggest meal at noon.** Noon is when Pitta is at its peak, and your agni is at its highest.

- ☐ **Eat in a quiet, settled environment.** Turn the TV off, put your smartphone down, and put other distractions away. If you're at work, step away from your desk and find a quiet spot to eat. Pleasant conversation and chit-chat are fine, but avoid stressful topics. Gently focus on your meal and hold gratitude for the ingredients and the chef. Again, if you're at work, avoid talking shop while you eat.

- ☐ **Don't eat on the go.** Sit down to eat your meals. Eating while standing or walking aggravates Vata dosha and leads to digestive upset. If possible, sit comfortably for a few minutes after finishing your meal to give your digestive juices a good start. Jumping up immediately after a meal can disrupt your digestion.

- ☐ **Avoid eating when angry, upset, or anxious.** Take a few deep breaths to calm your system so it's ready to receive food.

- ☐ **Avoid frozen foods**, overly processed foods (like boxed breakfast cereal—even when it's low in sugar), refined sugars and flours, and artificial foods, colors, and preservatives. These can all lead to a buildup of ama.

- ☐ **Do not to eat leftovers** for the same reason. Food should be freshly prepared whenever possible.

☐ **Do not heat honey**, whether by cooking, baking, or adding it to your hot tea. According to Ayurveda, honey becomes toxic when heated. If you like honey in your tea or coffee, wait until your beverage has cooled a bit.

☐ **Don't eat a large meal in the evening**, especially right before bed. At night, your body performs crucial rest-and-repair functions so you're ready to start the next day fresh. Give your body several hours to digest dinner before hitting the hay; otherwise, you'll burden your digestive system. If you are hungry before bed, drink a cup of warm milk to tide you over.

☐ **Sip warm water throughout the day** to keep your body's channels of purification clear. It's helpful to sip warm or room-temperature water during meals as well.

☐ **Keep your digestive fire kindled** by avoiding foods that dampen its flames, such as cold foods, ice-cold beverages, ice, leftover food, highly processed foods, frozen foods, or canned foods. These things can all lead to ama.

☐ **Take a short, gentle walk after meals** to boost digestion. But don't hop up right away! Sit for a few minutes to give your body time to start the digestive process.

Even if you incorporate only four or five of the above suggestions into your daily routine, you'll find that you improve your digestion, increase ojas, and decrease ama.

The Power of a Plant-Based Diet

You don't need to swear off eating all meat forever starting tomorrow. Start where you are right now and make little changes that can result in a big difference in how you feel. My big-city Chicago clients are meat eaters, vegetarians, vegans, Keto buffs, and everything in between. Whatever your daily diet looks like now, you can easily adapt what you're eating to be more in line with Ayurvedic principles.

That being said, traditional Ayurvedic doctors generally recommend a lacto-vegetarian diet rich in fresh produce and healthy fats. The reason is simple: a largely plant-based diet is easier to digest. Protein—your body's essential building blocks for muscles and organ tissue—is a vital component of the Ayurvedic diet. Instead of getting that protein from meats and fish, get it from legumes, nuts and seeds, and dairy, if your body tolerates it.

The Ayurvedic diet is somewhat similar to the vegan diet in its emphasis on plant-based nutrition, but while vegans favor raw food, Ayurveda recommends well-cooked and well-spiced veggies for optimal digestion.

The perception that vegetarians are thin, sickly looking, malnourished people is now a well-known fallacy. Legendary quarterback Tom Brady credits his largely vegan, low-carb diet for his success playing MVP-level football into his forties. Vegetarian tennis player Novak Djokovic won five Wimbledon titles while on a plant-based diet. Vegan bodybuilders attest that you don't need to eat beef to beef up.

The meat-alone-builds-muscle myth has long been exactly that—a myth in North America. Up until recently, the USDA promoted a Food Pyramid diagram that was out of date. Among other recommendations, the diagram encouraged six to eleven servings of bread, pasta, cereal, or rice daily (definitely a carbohydrate overload), classified all fats as bad (some fats are actually good for you), and lumped proteins like red meat and poultry together with nuts and legumes. The pyramid was replaced in 2011 by an improved plate diagram that reduced carbs and increased produce, but it still left a lot of questions unanswered about proteins, fats, and processed foods.

Today, scientists have discovered what Ayurveda has known all along: better health comes from a balanced, largely vegetarian diet that's rich in produce, fiber, and healthy fats like those from nuts and olive oil. In a 2014 *Annual Reviews* article, researchers at Yale University's Prevention Research Center concluded that "A diet of minimally processed foods close to nature, predominantly plants, is decisively associated with health promotion and disease prevention."

In keeping with Ayurvedic guidelines, the space on your plate at any given meal should be taken up by about 30% protein (from legumes, nuts, seeds, and dairy), 40% cooked vegetables, and 20% healthy grains. Does this sound like a heck of a lot of veggies? Consider this: fresh foods are rich in *prana*, the life-giving energy that fuels growth and nourishes your body. They're also abundant in vital nutrients and fiber which is needed to sweep your digestive tract clean.

If you feel that you're unable to go without meat at this time, take baby steps toward a more plant-based diet. Start by upping your intake of fresh produce, cutting back your intake of carbs, and eating organic, non-genetically modified meats. Favor lighter, more easily digested proteins like fish and poultry over heavier fare like red meat.

Eating Ayurvedically is about much more than just favoring a plant-based diet. It's also about eating according to your doshas.

Go organic. The texts of Ayurveda were recorded long before modern scientists began dousing produce with chemical pesticides or tampering with genetically modified organisms (GMOs). Foods that have been doused with inorganic fertilizers and sprays often contain toxic residue that can accumulate in your body. So, buy organic whenever possible.

How Diet Affects the Doshas

If you took the *What's My Dosha Quiz* in the introduction, you know your prakriti, or Ayurvedic mind-body type. This section will explore specific dietary guidelines for each dosha type.

Like increases like, and opposites attract. For example, if Pitta types, who have a lot of heat in their systems, regularly eat hot, spicy, or acidic foods, their emotions will flare up and become overheated. It will be difficult for them to become calm and relaxed, unless they are willing to change their diet to foods that help cool their emotions. As a Pitta type myself, I can personally attest to this wisdom; hot chili peppers send my temper through the roof.

"But what about my beloved spicy sriracha sauce?" you may protest. To that, I say, everything in moderation. If you're a Pitta type and you love spicy things, try not to eat hot, spicy foods too often. If you continue to eat acidic foods, you will increasingly notice things like skin irritations, stomach acidity, irritability, and other Pitta-related health problems.

Now, think of someone who often feels lethargic, depressed, and puts on weight easily. These people have lots of heavy, earthy Kapha energy. If such a person eats rich, oily foods and lots of sweets, they will only add more heaviness to their bodies and their emotions.

Similarly, a whirlwind Vata type who often feels cold and anxious would benefit from a steady diet of warm, grounding meals rather than raw foods eaten on the go.

These are just a few broad examples of how eating according to your dosha can make a big difference.

The Six Tastes and Their Influence on the Doshas

Taste is an important factor in eating Ayurvedically. You know how some foods make your mouth water, whereas others make you want to gag? That's because taste is actually the first step in digestion. When food tastes pleasant to the tongue, it encourages saliva production that's necessary to start breaking food down. We experience taste differently because that's where the doshas come in.

Some tastes increase certain doshas, whereas others decrease them. Ayurveda teaches that every type of food consists of a combination of the five basic elements of nature (earth, air, water, fire, and space). Each of these elements are present in the tastes, and they have a direct impact on the doshas.

Here's a list of tastes and how they affect the doshas:

Sweet

Sweet foods have earth and water elements. Therefore, they increase Kapha and decrease Vata and Pitta. Some examples include rice, milk, sweet fruits, bread, sugar, peppermint, licorice root, dates, figs, and pasta.

Sour

Sour foods have earth and fire elements. Therefore, they increase Pitta and Kapha and decrease Vata. Some examples include lemon, yogurt, sour fruits, cheese, green grapes, and tamarind.

Salty

Salty foods have water and fire elements. Therefore, they increase Pitta and Kapha and decrease Vata. Some examples include salt, which can be added to any food, and seaweed.

Bitter

Bitter foods have air and space elements. Therefore, they increase Vata and decrease Pitta and Kapha. Some examples include turmeric, leafy greens, fenugreek seeds, and aloe vera.

Pungent

Pungent foods have air and fire elements. Therefore, they increase Vata and Pitta and decrease Kapha. Some examples include ginger, onion, garlic, hing (asafoetida), pepper, and radish.

Astringent

Astringent foods have air and earth elements. Therefore, they increase Vata and decrease Kapha and Pitta. Some examples include lentils, beans, and quinoa, as well as apple, pomegranate, and unripe bananas.

According to Ayurveda, to keep the doshas balanced, have a bit of each of the six tastes in each meal. You can use the examples above as a general guide or simply use Ayurvedic *churna* (dosha-specific spice mixtures that include all six tastes). You can mix up your own or buy prepared churnas from MAPI (https://www.mapi.com).

While it's helpful to engage the six tastes in each meal, it's even more important to eat according to your dosha type when possible. However, it's also important to understand the three different qualities of foods—sattva, rajas, and tamas.

The Three Universal Qualities: Sattva, Rajas, and Tamas

You've just learned how taste affects digestion and how different foods impact the doshas. Now, let's discuss the subtle qualities of food—and how those qualities impact your digestion and well-being.

According to Ayurvedic texts, everything in the universe and in individuals is comprised of three universal qualities. These are known as the three *gunas*: sattva, rajas, and tamas. These qualities permeate all of life; in fact, there would be no creation, no life as we know it, without the three gunas. Ancient Ayurvedic texts categorize all types of food into one of three categories: sattvic, rajasic, and tamasic.

Sattva

Sattva is the quality of purity, harmony, and balance. It is the universal quality of life that nurtures. When you have a lot of ojas in your system, it leads to a sattvic mind and heart. A person that we may call highly sattvic will be calm, peaceful, loving, and have the ability to uplift all those around them. Sattvic people tend to be positive, wise, and noble.

Sattvic Foods

In Ayurveda, certain foods are said to promote the quality of sattva in the mind, body, and heart. These foods are sweet, calming, and fortifying by nature. Sattvic foods include rice, wheat, mung beans and other legumes, most dairy products (such as paneer, a fresh soft cheese, and boiled milk with spices, but not aged cheeses and homogenized or pasteurized products), fresh vegetables (well cooked), fresh fruits, ghee, blanched almonds or almond milk, some nuts (walnuts, pecans, brazil nuts, pine nuts, pistachios, and chestnuts), and some seeds (pumpkin, sesame, sunflower, and flax).

Rajas

Rajas is the quality of action, passion, and movement. Rajas is what spurs on sattva and propels creation itself. In the individual, rajas leads to motion, dynamism, and energy. However, if a person has an excess of rajas in their system, they can become restless, irritable, unhappy, and overly stimulated.

Rajasic Foods

Foods that are rajasic have their place; they can bring dynamism and stimulation. Eaten in excess, they can lead to restlessness, hyperactivity, hyperacidity, and overly aroused passions. Rajasic foods tend toward the addictive side (think French fries and cola beverages); once you start eating them, it's hard to kick the habit or exercise self-restraint. Rajasic foods include garlic, onion, coffee and other caffeinated drinks, alcohol, highly spiced or salted foods, and fried foods. Fish and chicken are rajasic, too, but can be eaten in moderation.

Tamas

Tamas is the quality of inertia, heaviness, and destruction. At first, this guna may sound negative to you, but growth comes from destroying the old to make way for something new and more evolutionary, just as fungi help to decompose fallen trees in the forest. In the individual, some tamas is inevitable (think of your body's natural waste systems), but an excess of this heavy, lethargic energy isn't great for your health.

Tamasic Foods

Tamasic foods increase inertia, laziness, and dull minds. They're best eaten in limited quantities—especially when you're feeling under the weather. Tamasic foods include mushrooms, some fermented foods (like vinegar or stale leftovers), refined flours and sugars, frozen foods, canned foods, aged cheeses, overly processed foods, heavier meats (like red meat), and processed meats (like canned meat or sausage).

While sattva is certainly the more admirable guna—and the one many hope will increasingly dominate in society—small amounts of rajas and tamas are required to support and uphold sattva.

History has repeatedly shown that in times of societal injustice, some level of upheaval and destruction is necessary before a more peaceful and just era can emerge. Similarly, our bodies sometimes seem to revolt against us and produce symptoms of discomfort and dis-ease, spurring us on to find new ways to purify and restore greater balance and health.

Every recommendation in this book will lead you naturally in the direction of more and more sattva in your diet and your life.

Say no to GMOs. Genetically modified foods are created by splicing the genes of one organism (such as a fish) into another organism (such as a tomato). The far-ranging implications of engineered foods aren't known at this point, but it's not scientifically certain they are safe to consume. Ayurveda places a strong emphasis on foods that are rich in *chetana*, nature's intelligence. Since certified organic foods do not contain GMOs, favor organic whenever possible.

A Guide to Eating for Your Dosha

Below is some basic information on how to eat according to your dosha. If you scored mostly Vata on the quiz, follow the Vata diet; if you scored mostly Pitta, follow the Pitta diet, and so on.

If one dosha, however, was just a little bit higher than another, you should balance both. For instance, if you are mostly Vata, with just a little less Pitta, eat warming foods to pacify Vata's cooling influence while keeping in mind not to overheat Pitta. In the chilly winter months, that balance will be easier to strike. In summer months, pay closer attention to Pitta's heating influence.

Vata-Balancing Diet

Vata is cool, dry, light, and irregular by nature. To bring this dosha into balance, eat things that are warm, moist, well-cooked, and grounding. Think hearty, well-spiced soups and stews rather than cold, raw foods like salads and crudités, which can aggravate Vata.

Because Vata is erratic by nature, Vata people benefit whenever routine is introduced. If you're a Vata type, eat three meals each day around the same time. Dieting, portion control, fasting, and skipping meals are all things that will throw Vata types off balance. On the other hand, you can generally get away with eating larger quantities of food, so long as you digest them well.

Sample Daily Diet for Vata

Breakfast: Warm cooked gluten-free cereal, or gluten-free toast with sugar-free jam and sunflower seed butter

Snack: A handful of almonds or walnuts

Noon: A warm, cooked meal. Make lunch your biggest meal of the day.

Afternoon: Low-sugar protein shake

Dinner: A warm, filling soup or stew

Before Bed: Hot milk, if needed

Tastes	**Favor/increase**: Sweet, salty, sour **Avoid/reduce**: Bitter, pungent, astringent
Fruit	**Favor/increase**: Sweet fruits, such as grapes, cherries, melons, avocados, coconuts, pomegranates, mangos, and sweet, fully ripened oranges, pineapples, and plums **Avoid/reduce**: Sour fruits such as grapefruits, olives, papayas, and unripe pineapples and plums
Vegetables	**Favor/increase**: Asparagus, cucumbers, potatoes, sweet potatoes, green leafy vegetables, pumpkins, broccoli, cauliflower, celery, okra, lettuce, green beans, and zucchini **Avoid/reduce**: Hot peppers, tomatoes, carrots, beets, onions, garlic, radishes, and spinach
Grains	**Favor/increase**: Rice, wheat, couscous **Avoid/reduce**: Barley, corn, millet, buckwheat, rye, and oats
Protein	**Avoid/reduce**: All beans, except for tofu and mung dal. All nuts are good.
Spices	**Favor/increase**: Cardamom, cumin, ginger, cinnamon, salt, cloves, mustard seed, and small quantities of black pepper
Oils	**Favor/increase**: All oils are good for balancing Vata
Dairy	**Favor/increase**: All dairy products, if tolerated. Always boil milk before you drink it. Drink milk warm. Don't drink milk with a full meal.
Sweeteners	**Favor/increase**: All sweeteners are good (in moderation) for pacifying Vata.

Pitta-Balancing Diet

Pitta is fiery, oily, intense, and sharp by nature. To bring this dosha into balance, eat cooling, sweet, and relatively dry foods that prevent Pitta from overheating. Think avocado toast and pasta with fresh veggies rather than spicy curries and deep-fried foods. Increase your intake of sweet, bitter, and astringent tastes while cutting back on pungent, sour, and salty tastes. Although Pitta types are sometimes drawn to hot, spicy, and oily foods like curries, avoid them.

Because Pitta's digestive fires are naturally strong, feed them regularly. Pitta people should never skip meals, lest they become hangry. Many Pitta types are physically active as well, so they need solid, balanced meals to fuel their adventures.

Sample Daily Diet for Pitta

Breakfast: Cooked cereal (like oatmeal) with soaked figs, raisins, or dates, plus blanched almonds and walnuts

Snack: Piece of sweet, juicy fruit, if needed

Noon: A warm, cooked meal with equal portions of a grain like rice, a protein like lentils or chicken, and a generous helping of freshly cooked veggies. Avocados at lunch are great for Pitta types. Their fiery appetites can also handle a small salad with some cooling cucumbers (raw foods are generally not advised for other dosha types).

Pitta's craving for protein can be satisfied by adding more nuts and seeds to a dish. Too much meat consumption can be heating for Pitta, so avoid having it every day. Make lunch your biggest meal of the day. Satisfy your sweet tooth with a fresh fruit cobbler.

Afternoon: Almond milk with blanched almonds and a few dates would be excellent as a snack for energy in the afternoon after your lunch has digested.

Dinner: Same as lunch except less protein and no nuts or seeds. Your plate should be 60% vegetables, 30% grains and 10% protein.

Before Bed: Hot milk, if needed

Tastes	**Favor/increase**: Sweet, bitter, astringent **Avoid/reduce**: Salty, sour, pungent
Fruit	**Favor/increase**: Sweet fruits, such as grapes, cherries, melons, avocados, coconuts, pomegranates, mangos, and sweet, fully ripened oranges, pineapples, and plums **Avoid/reduce**: Sour fruits such as grapefruits, olives, papayas, and unripe pineapples and plums
Vegetables	**Favor/increase**: Asparagus, cucumbers, potatoes, sweet potatoes, green leafy vegetables, pumpkins, broccoli, cauliflower, celery, okra, green beans, and zucchini **Avoid/reduce**: Hot peppers, tomatoes, carrots, beets, onions, garlic, radishes, and spinach
Grains	**Favor/increase**: Rice **Avoid/reduce**: Millet
Protein	**Favor/increase**: Lentils, legumes, and lean protein like chicken **Avoid/reduce**: Fish, especially at night
Spices	**Favor/increase**: Cinnamon, coriander, cardamom, and fennel. Fresh ginger is okay in small amounts. **Avoid/reduce**: Powdered ginger, cumin, fenugreek, black pepper, clove, celery seed, salt, and mustard seed. Chili peppers and cayenne should be avoided entirely.
Oils	**Favor/increase**: Olive, sunflower, and coconut oils **Avoid/reduce**: Sesame, almond, and corn oil
Dairy	**Favor/increase**: Milk, butter, and ghee **Avoid/reduce**: Reduce yogurt, cheese, sour cream, and cultured buttermilk (their sour tastes aggravate Pitta). Yogurt in the form of lassi is okay.

Sweeteners	**Favor/increase**: Most sweeteners are good in moderation.
	Avoid/reduce: Honey and molasses

Kapha-Balancing Diet

Kapha is slow, moist, and oily by nature. To bring this dosha type into balance, spice things up! Eat a variety of fresh, healthy, and well-spiced meals. Think colorful veggie curries and stir-fries, rather than fettucine alfredo and creamy cakes. Eating vegetables is particularly beneficial for Kaphas, who tend toward sluggish digestion.

Because Kapha types tend to gain weight easily, they should eat lighter portions—and cut down on desserts. Rich, creamy, sweet, and heavy foods might appeal to Kaphas (they usually love bread, butter, cookies, donuts, and potato chips), but those foods can weigh them down and lead to further inertia. Kaphas can be susceptible to gluten intolerance, which is why I often recommend they go gluten-free.

Kapha types should avoid eating a lot of food at one time and should leave at least three hours between meals. Snacking isn't recommended, other than a piece of ripe fruit or a low-sugar protein shake.

Sample Daily Diet for Kapha

Breakfast: Stewed fruit. Can add a few almonds or walnuts (soaked overnight for optimal absorption) if more substance is needed.

Snack: Piece of ripe fruit, if needed

Noon: A warm, cooked meal with a lean protein (such as lentils or fish), a small portion of grains (such as buckwheat), and a large quantity of cooked leafy greens and other mixed vegetables. A good 50% of your plate should be covered in veggies. The bitter taste of leafy greens works wonders to reduce cravings for sugar and salt. Make lunch your biggest meal of the day.

Afternoon: Low-sugar protein shake

Dinner: A light soup or stew

Before Bed: Hot milk if needed

Tastes	**Favor/increase**: Bitter, pungent, astringent **Avoid/reduce**: Sweet, salty, sour
Fruit	**Favor/increase**: Lighter fruits, such as apples and pears **Avoid/reduce**: Heavy or sour fruits, such as oranges, bananas, pineapples, figs, dates, avocados, coconuts, and melons
Vegetables	**Favor/increase:** All are fine, especially leafy greens **Avoid/reduce:** Tomatoes, cucumbers, sweet potatoes, and zucchini
Grains	**Favor/increase**: Most grains are fine, especially barley, millet, and buckwheat. **Avoid/reduce**: Too much wheat, oats, or rice
Protein	**Favor/increase**: Legumes, lean protein like chicken or fish **Avoid/reduce**: Red meats, soy, eggs
Spices	**Favor/increase**: All are fine except for salt, which must be used in moderation (salt increases Kapha).
Oils	**Favor/increase**: Olive oil, ghee in small amounts **Avoid/reduce**: Most oils are too heavy, especially butter and coconut oil in winter months or cooler climates
Dairy	**Favor/increase**: Low-fat milk is best or dilute whole milk with water. Always boil milk before you drink it—which makes it easier to digest—and drink it warm. Do not take milk with a full meal or with sour or salty food. You can add one or two pinches of turmeric or ginger to whole milk before boiling to

	reduce any Kapha-increasing qualities in the milk. A teaspoon of yogurt or diluted lassi at lunch is okay. **Avoid/reduce:** aged cheese, no cheese at night
Sweeteners	**Favor/increase**: Honey in moderation is excellent for reducing Kapha. Stevia is also good. **Avoid/reduce:** Most other sweeteners

Ayurvedic Portion Size: Most of us eat a little more than we actually need to. According to Ayurveda, the ideal portion size at any given meal is whatever will fit into your two cupped hands.

Another helpful tip: Eat until just before you feel full (or you've eaten to about 3/4 of your capacity). If you're burping, that's a sign that it's time to stop. The way most of us eat on Thanksgiving is way beyond the recommended Ayurvedic portion size.

Chapter 3: Sleep

Sleep Is a Beautiful Thing

Sleep is a beautiful thing, but most people don't get enough. Millions of American adults, teenagers and even small children have trouble sleeping. The main reason is anxiety or stress. Other reasons for lack of sleep could be diet and lifestyle choices.

Whatever the reason for not sleeping well, whether you're not able to fall asleep or you wake up often in the middle of the night, here are the best sleep recommendations that will having you sleeping like a baby and waking up feeling fresh and ready to go.

People often claim to be night people, not morning people. Unless you work the night shift, you've created yourself to be a night person by your lifestyle decisions. You may think that you are getting eight hours of sleep, so it shouldn't really matter when you go to bed, but that's simply not the case. Medical experts advocate an early bedtime and getting seven to eight hours of sleep. Children and teenagers usually need more sleep, around nine to eleven hours.

Staying up late is unhealthy; it will impact your health over time. You don't have to be in bed by 8:00 p.m., but be in bed by 10:00 p.m. or 11:00 p.m. at the latest. If you stay up later, you will catch a second wind which will make falling asleep harder.

Ayurveda says that being asleep by 10:00 p.m. helps the efficiency of the metabolic processes that occur between 10:00 p.m. and 2:00 a.m. that night. The nutrients you consumed during the day will get assimilated and used for fuel the next day. By missing this opportunity, your digestion can be ruined. If you start getting to bed earlier, there will be a noticeable increase in the quality of your life.

Recommendations for Getting a Better Night's Sleep

Transcendental Meditation

Learn the Transcendental Meditation technique. I've seen the fastest results with this one thing alone for better sleep.

Here is one person's story on how TM helped her with her decade-long sleep problems:

"Before learning the TM technique, I tried everything natural and unnatural to get to sleep. Even medications did not work that well and, even if they did sometimes help, they made me feel groggy. I was exhausted all the time and would drag through the day using caffeine just to stay awake and focused, so I didn't lose my job. The lack of sleep caused weight gain, memory problems, and mood swings. I was unhappy and would snap at people for no reason, which almost cost me my job since one of those people was my boss. I knew I had to get a handle on things.

"One day after learning the TM technique, I slept through the night and like magic it's been keeping me asleep most nights. If I wake up to use the rest room, I go right back to sleep. Although I felt great and more refreshed after the first night of a better sleep, now after doing TM for over a year it's been a huge transformation in my life. My relationships have improved, and people are noticing. There is no longer the need to use food or caffeine to excess to stay awake or quell my stress. I feel back to myself again. I started losing weight and have enough energy now to exercise and make better food choices."

Here's another client's story. As he traveled around, a pharmaceutical representative expressed his inability to sleep to the people he befriended. They were all too happy to help him out by providing him with free samples of all the latest sleep drugs. They gave these pills away to him like candy. Before he knew it, he was on three different sleep meds—horse pills, he called them. He was taking up to six or seven of each. The more he used, the more he needed to get proper sleep. He built up such a resistance to them he needed more and more.

Even with all the pills, he was still not falling asleep until 4:00 a.m. These medications messed up his sleep cycle, so he started sleeping most of the day and staying up late. Eventually he recognized the negative side effects on his body. The pills were affecting his gut health; he gained weight and became a diabetic.

Once he changed his diet and lifestyle, he did much better. He learned TM, which was a great beginning, and implemented many Ayurveda recommendations for sleep. It took him many months of small changes to reach his goals. But, if you are dealing with a problem that took decades to create, it can take time to heal.

Lights Out by 9:45 p.m.

Early to bed and early to rise makes a man healthy, wealthy, and wise. That expression may be a bit of a stretch, since you may not see your bank account grow overnight; however, health is wealth. If you are a night owl, it may be hard to go to bed early right away. Start by shifting your bedtime 15 minutes earlier each night until you reach that goal of 10:00 p.m. If you are out late due to travel or the occasional event, no worries. Just get back on track again. Try for this bedtime most nights.

If you have work you need to do, you will eventually start waking up earlier, so essentially you won't be losing any hours.

Eat Better

Don't eat dinner too late at night, or graze later in the evening. It's sad that people get in the habit of eating late at night. That can cause terrible sleep, resulting in bad dreams or tossing and turning all night.

The types of food you eat can cause stomach acidity, which is another reason for poor sleep. Eat dinner at least three hours before getting to bed. If you are hungry several hours after dinner, drink warm cow's, rice, hemp, oat, or almond milk. Implementing a better diet for your body type should help as well.

Exercise

Don't exercise too late at night. Exercise or yoga during the day, however, will promote better sleep at night. A brisk thirty-minute walk as well as yoga and strength training will make you want to crawl into bed by 10:00 p.m.

Reduce Electronics

Reduce your use of cellphones, computers, and TV before bed. One important rule: Don't sleep with your cellphone or Wi-Fi on. These disrupt sleep and are among the top reasons why most people don't sleep well. Many people still put their cellphones under their pillows or on the night table. That's way too close.

Switch your cellphones to airplane mode or, better yet, turn them off completely if you want better sleep at night as well as better focus the next day.

Oil Massage

To relax, put warm oil on your head and feet, and then place a towel on the pillow and old socks on your feet. Oil is very calming. You can do a full oil massage and warm bath with Epsom salts and a splash of lavender oil.

Herbal Tea, etc.

If you are having a hard time sleeping, try herbal remedies. For example, drink Vata herbal tea, which is very calming. Or try some *Stress Free Mind* tablets from MAPI.com. Take two tablets twice a day after breakfast and dinner and another two before bed.

Take a small amount of melatonin, depending upon your body size and how you react to it. Some people don't do well with melatonin. If that's you, stick with the *Stress Free Mind* tablets.

Chapter 4: Movement, Yoga, and Exercise

Everyone knows that for optimal health, they need to move their bodies more. Nonetheless, many people are not getting the exercise they need. Doctors now claim that sitting is the new smoking. What they mean is that if you are sitting all day long at your job, it is equivalent to being a heavy smoker in terms of the negative effects on your health. If you are not already exercising regularly, get motivated.

As with starting a new diet, being regular with exercise can be difficult. Energy is the biggest factor for people. That is why I recommend exercise in the morning for all body types. Ayurveda says that the best time for exercise is either 6:00 to 10:00 a.m. or 6:00 to 10:00 p.m., so you can choose later at night if you need to as long as it doesn't get you too revved up so you can't fall asleep. If you need to exercise at night due to your work schedule or other reasons, do it earlier, like 6:00 or 7:00 p.m. Just don't eat too much after the exercise, since eating too late at night is not good for you.

Since the type of yoga I recommend is settling, it can be done any time of day, even before bed. The same guidelines for exercise in terms of when to eat also apply to yoga. Do not perform yoga positions on a full stomach, and wait at least half an hour after a snack.

Timing Exercise and Yoga

What is the best time to exercise in relationship to eating, meditating, and sleeping? Because it's good to eat something after you exercise, you can meditate, exercise, and then eat breakfast (if your morning routine allows it). Or you can meditate, eat breakfast, digest a little, and then exercise. The same schedule would apply to the evening. Do not eat a huge breakfast if you're going to exercise a half hour later. A smaller meal or snack is better. After a large meal, wait at least an hour or two for digestion before exercising.

Don't exercise when you are hungry or not well-hydrated. In warmer climates and seasons, you need natural sugars such as fruit, fresh juices, or coconut water to replace your electrolytes, especially if exercise induces a lot of sweating. Exercising in the morning without eating may work if you are not awake too many hours prior to doing it. However, if you fast and then try to exercise before lunch, you may feel weak. So, if you haven't eaten for many hours, it's best to have some fruit or a small snack half an hour or an hour before your exercise.

Never exercise at noon if you've only eaten a piece of fruit or something light. This can cause low blood sugar and a feeling of not being grounded mentally. If such Vata vitiation happens, it defeats the purpose of exercising and following health recommendations.

Don't fast for sixteen to seventeen hours, which Ayurveda would not recommend unless you are a Kapha type and extremely overweight. Even then, it's not something I would encourage. The daily fasting Ayurveda recommends is to eat your dinner by 6:00 or 7:00 p.m. and then eat your breakfast between 6:00 and 9:00 a.m. Then you would have fasted for twelve to fifteen hours, and that's enough.

If you skip breakfast and do not eat until noon or later, this is not good. Over the long term, this can be unhealthy for most people. If you eat too much food late at night, you will not be hungry until noon since the evening food sat in your stomach and didn't get properly digested.

Why Exercise and Do Yoga?

If you know the benefits of exercise and yoga, it will keep you motivated to do them.

- ☐ Improves mood
- ☐ Reduces anxiety, depression, and lack of motivation
- ☐ Raises self-esteem
- ☐ Provides mental and physical energy

- ☐ Increases focus
- ☐ Improves metabolism for better digestion and weight management.
- ☐ Strengthens joints and keeps them flexible and strong.
- ☐ Improves heart health
- ☐ Reduces the risk of certain cancers

Below are my recommendations for exercise and yoga for different doshas or body types.

Vata Types

True Vata types, who are very thin with small bones, do better with less intensive aerobics, although everyone needs to get their heart rate up. My suggestion for Vata types is fast walking, but for a shorter duration than for Pitta and Kapha types. Vata types can also enjoy swimming, biking, dancing, and other activities, but not for extended periods, especially if they are very thin. Vata types, if they are very thin, need to worry about losing too much weight. If they are interested in gaining weight, they should do more Pilates and weight training. They may also need an exercise and yoga buddy, if they are not good with being regular with exercise.

If you are a Vata type and a good athlete, you will be good at sprinting in track, tennis, and anything that requires a thin physique and being able to move quickly. Most Vata types can move at swift speeds, but if they don't have support from some Pitta and Kapha qualities in their constitution, they may not have stamina.

Michael Phelps is a great example of a true Vata type. Note that any person who is very tall or very short has substantial Vata in their constitution. Phelps epitomizes the quick Vata nature by setting so many world records for being the fastest swimmer. Similarly, Shelly-Ann Fraser-Pryce is the fastest woman sprinter in the world. When you look at men or women who are sprinters, they have a thin small frame. By having less weight, they move more quickly.

Kapha types, on the other hand, could not compete in the area of sprinting, especially if they are built like a football player. Pitta types, however, can be good runners if they have some Vata.

Why too much exercise is not good for Vata types

If Vata types are physically fit and occasionally go for a two-hour hike and are sore the next day, that is not a problem. However, two-hour workouts several times a week is another story. I don't recommend a two-hour daily workout for anyone unless they are a professional athlete.

Here is a story of what not to do:

One of my clients went for a bike ride for two hours straight before meeting me. He was feeling proud that he went extremely fast in the wind and hot sun non-stop. Anyone would have been able to tell that he was totally disoriented afterward. This is the negative effect of too much exercise. The wind and fast movement vitiate Vata dosha.

Exercise that can be so good can have a negative side effect. In this case, his bike ride affected his mental well-being. He is a small-boned Vata type with little meat on him. I suspect he didn't eat much before the bike ride, and that made it worse. He seemed to like to do this quite often, probably because it's exhilarating on one level, but he didn't understand the long-term debilitating effects.

Pure Vata types often skip meals and then feel unsettled, which is the opposite effect that exercise should have. My client was probably dehydrated from being in the hot sun for so long. He should drink coconut water or other electrolytes after a workout especially in warm weather.

Moderate exercise relaxes and soothes Vata's anxiety and worry, but too much can increase these negative emotions.

Vata Type recommendations for exercise and yoga

☐ **Aerobic** exercise for 20 to 25 minutes, 4 to 5 days per week.

☐ **Strength training** 3 to 4 times a week for about 20 minutes with lighter weights since the smaller bones of Vatas can't handle too much weight.

☐ **Daily yoga** for 10 to 15 minutes once or twice a day. Those who are trained in the TM technique can learn yoga with their TM teacher. It's more practical to do yoga at home so you can fit it in more often. If not, any type of gentle yoga that is offered at a studio or online is fine.

□ **Pilates** is good because it involves stretching and slower movements good for Vata dosha.

Pitta Types

Pitta types tend to be the most regular exercisers. Most top athletes have strong Pitta qualities in their constitution. They have so much drive to compete and be the best. If they also have Kapha for stamina and Vata for quickness, they really excel. Of course, some genetics for athleticism is crucial for any professional athlete. One needs excellent coordination and an adeptness at a particular sport as well as the discipline to practice, practice, practice. Pittas, who are often type A personalities, can possess good discipline.

Although Pitta types can handle more exercise than a pure Vata type, they do need to be careful not to overdo it as well. All body types need to keep exercise to a minimum. If you are not an athlete, then thirty to forty minutes of aerobic exercise is enough for a Pitta type; otherwise, just for good health twenty to thirty minutes is sufficient. It's your choice.

If a child or teenager is a Pitta type, this recommendation varies. A child or teenager in organized sports will be doing more, but if your child is not in a sport, then you need to see they are getting enough exercise: at least four to five times a week of thirty minutes of a sport, brisk walk, or other physical movement.

True Pitta athletes would include Lindsey Vonn, the former World Cup alpine ski racer, or many famous mountain climbers. Also, aggressive sports like football favor Pitta types. Of course, anyone playing a sport has some level of Pitta dosha.

Sometimes you don't need much Pitta, since the Kapha types enjoy the comradery of organized sports. Pittas can do sports that are single events and not necessarily group oriented. They sometimes enjoy being on their own—as with skiers, mountain climbers, and triathletes.

Pitta types are fearless risk takers. If this happens to be you or one of your children, you need to understand that Pitta types love to push themselves beyond their limit to be the best. A pure Vata type can't relate to that since they would not have the courage or drive to do sports where there is risk of injury. For example, they may not like skiing because it requires them to be up at great heights; they usually have too much fear for that.

Pitta Type recommendations for exercise and yoga

- ☐ **Aerobic** type exercise for 25 to 35 minutes, 4 to 5 days per week.

- ☐ **Strength training** 3 to 4 times a week for about 20 minutes with medium weights. Your bones are stronger than a pure Vata, but still not as strong as a Kapha, so be careful.

- ☐ **Daily yoga** for 10 to 15 minutes, once or twice a day. Those who are trained in the TM technique can learn this yoga with their TM teacher. It's more practical to do yoga at home so you can fit it in more often. If not, any type of gentle yoga that is offered at a studio or online is fine.

- ☐ **Pilates** is good because it involves a lot of stretching. Sometimes slower movements are good for a Pitta's aggressive nature.

Kapha Types

If an individual is a Pitta-Kapha type, they will be most successful in sports. They have the drive of Pitta and the stamina of Kapha. You see this with athletes who have to play four to six hours of tennis nonstop or with triathletes who have to run, bike, or swim for many hours. Those with a strong physiology have an advantage.

An individual with Kapha predominance, however, will not want to be regular with exercise and yoga, even though they need it the most. Some Kapha types end up doing sports like tennis, volleyball, or anything where they don't have to move too much if they don't want to. Kaphas on a subtle level learn early on how to hit with power and precision so the return ball doesn't make them run around the court. I watched Serena Williams in her later years change her strategy when she would get more winded, so she didn't have to move as much—and it worked.

Many tennis players can win the game with a powerful serve that can't be returned by their opponent. Serena has so much physical strength and skill that she learned to be more efficient in her game to exert the least amount of effort, which is necessary as athletes age and still want to compete.

Even though he doesn't appear to be a big Kapha type, Roger Federer has a calm demeanor. He doesn't expend energy by getting mad and all worked up during a match. That gives him more stamina.

Worry, anxiety, and anger can dissipate physical and mental energy. Kaphas can stay emotionally more balanced for longer periods of time and have a reserve of energy that pure Vata and Pitta types don't have. It's like money in the bank for them as athletes that they can cash in as needed.

The average person, who is not a professional athlete or has not been regular with exercise throughout their life, truly needs exercise the most. When Kapha dosha is out of balance, they get depressed and unmotivated. Exercise helps with both of these situations, but how do you get motivated if you suffer from this? First, find an early morning meditation buddy or an online class that serves as a buddy. Meditation will give you more motivation and energy. Then commit to thirty to forty-five minutes of exercise. If you prefer fast walking and the weather is nice, do that. Treadmills are great for the winter months.

Since pure Kaphas can dread exercise, they should live with a Pitta type who can motivate and encourage them—even if they have to put them in front of a TV with a treadmill and their favorite TV show. Whatever it takes to get the body moving.

This is what I have done with my husband, Bolton, who actually was a fantastic tennis player and athlete all his life. He swam as a teenager, and his family always plays tennis and badminton, takes long walks, and do other group activities when they get together. Even though they are now between fifty-five and sixty-five, they continue these health traditions. It's really impressive.

When they come to town, my husband will play these sports, but being the Kapha type he is, he won't initiate these activities on his own. He won't exercise regularly unless I push him. When I broke my ankle and couldn't work out, he didn't either. He joked that with the emotional trauma over my broken ankle, he needed to take a break.

If this sounds like you or someone you know, change this pattern. You won't regret it. Create a calendar of the days and time you will exercise, and keep with that schedule. You will need to do this at least five times per week. Even a brisk walk is good enough. Regularity is the key.

Kapha Type recommendations for exercise and yoga

- ☐ **Aerobic** exercise 30 to 40 minutes, 4 to 5 days per week. If you need to lose weight, then 40 minutes is better. A brisk walk is great or anything where your heart rate goes up and your body is moving. If you are a slender Kapha type, then 30 minutes is fine. Some people have the mental Kapha mindset and characteristics but are not necessarily overweight (if they are balanced).

- ☐ **Strength training** 3 to 4 times a week for about 20 minutes. Do what you can handle, and increase training time as you grow stronger. You want to keep your good muscle structure intact as you age, so you can lift groceries and stay strong.

- ☐ **Daily yoga** for 10 minutes, once or twice a day. Those who are trained in the TM technique can learn this yoga with their TM teacher. It's more practical to do yoga at home so you can fit it in more often. If not, any type of gentle yoga that is offered at a studio or online is fine.

- ☐ **Pilates** is good because it involves stretching, which is good for all types but especially for Kaphas who may not be as flexible. Anyone who sits all day can use Pilates.

Breath (Pranayama)

Pranayama is a breathing exercise from Ayurveda. Pranayama means "regulating the breath." The purpose of this exercise is to bring balance to both your mind and body through the flow of air through your body. It very naturally settles down your mind and physiology.

There are many types of pranayama, but the most practical and effective to begin with is the *alternate nostril breathing exercise*, which is simply alternating your breathing between your right and left nostrils. Practicing this exercise on a regular basis helps to open up and unblock channels in your physiology as the oxygen is circulated more thoroughly throughout your lungs and body.

In terms of the doshas, this exercise helps to balance Vata dosha. Since Vata dosha is the top dosha, this exercise balances all of the doshas.

Some of the specific benefits of pranayama are:

- ☐ Calms the mind
- ☐ Balances the nervous system

☐ Improves asthma conditions

☐ Balances the adrenal glands

Here are step-by-step instructions on how to practice this pranayama technique:

1. Sit upright in a quiet environment without any distractions. Sit without your legs being crossed, so you don't block any pathways in your body. If the weather is nice, you can sit near an open window and let in fresh air as long as it's not noisy outside. Close your eyes.

2. Start with your right hand, using your thumb on your right nostril and your middle and ring fingers on your left nostril. Begin by blocking the air flow in your right nostril by pressing your right thumb against the nostril. With your right nostril blocked, inhale slowly, easily, and softly through your left nostril. Continue inhaling until you can't inhale anymore. There is a point where you will know you can't take in more air.

3. Then take your right middle and ring finger and place them over your left nostril to block it. At the same time, release your thumb from your right nostril (unblocking the right nostril) and start exhaling the air you took in from your left nostril to flow out of your right nostril. Slowly, softly, exhale until your breath is out. Then begin inhaling into your right nostril again.

4. The main point is that after you start the first inhalation through your left nostril, continue through each nostril: exhale, inhale, switch nostrils, and so on.

5. Do this for five minutes twice a day. If you have learned the TM technique, do pranayama before your TM practice. If you are also doing yoga, the sequence for practice should be: yoga, pranayama, meditation.

Yoga Asanas

Ayurveda offers a physical exercise called *yoga asanas*, which are specific poses that develop flexibility and strength for your physiology. When people use the term *yoga*, they often mean practicing poses for flexibility and strength. However, there are many variations of these yoga exercises.

The yoga practice I recommend is Maharishi Yoga Asanas, which comes from Ayurveda and which emphasizes the development of greater balance of mind and body. Maharishi Yoga Asanas bring the awareness of the practitioner to a more unbounded state. It's not just about developing physical flexibility and strength; it's also about bringing your mind to a more settled, more balanced, more blissful state.

My yoga students prefer Maharishi Yoga Asanas to other yoga classes they have taken. Why? Because they experience a level of silence, or transcending, while practicing these asanas, which they did not experience in other yoga classes.

The guiding principle of Maharishi Yoga Asanas is to do exercises in an easy, effortless, gentle way at a slow pace, by practicing in silence and not straining. Maharishi Yoga Asanas have a particular sequence of poses designed to develop maximum flexibility, strength, and nourishment for your entire physiology.

The benefits of Maharishi Yoga Asanas that people notice include:

- ☐ Improved flexibility
- ☐ Normalized body weight
- ☐ Reduced high blood pressure
- ☐ Increased physical fitness
- ☐ Improved digestion
- ☐ Reduced back pain
- ☐ Improved circulation
- ☐ Improved organ health

Practice Maharishi Yoga Asanas twice a day for ten to fifteen minutes each time. If you are practicing Transcendental Meditation, practice Maharishi Yoga Asanas before each meditation.

To ensure you learn the poses correctly and gain the maximum benefit, it's best to learn these asanas from a certified teacher.

For more information and guidance, see https://www.miu.edu/yoga.

Chapter 5: Living with Nature's Rhythms

There's no denying that nature's rhythms influence our mental and physiological functioning. When the sun sets at night, we begin to feel sleepy. When the sun rises with the birds in the morning, we rouse from our slumber. The *sleep-wake cycle* is the most basic pattern in our circadian rhythms, which are governed by the body's internal clock. In that same way, we are also influenced by nature's seasons—we're chillier during winter, and we bask in the sun during summer.

When you're in tune with nature's rhythms, you tend to feel better. Have you ever pulled an all-nighter and then tried to function coherently the next day? If so, you know exactly what I'm talking about! In our fast-paced world, so many of us have learned to tune out our inner clock, ignoring our body's hunger signals and skipping meals, or staying up late on our smartphones when we're really craving a nourishing, fortifying night's sleep.

From the perspective of Ayurveda, the state of health and wholeness comes from living in alignment with the rhythms of nature—that is, following a lifestyle and diet that promote balance throughout the day. As you'll see in this chapter, those natural rhythms have a lot to do with the doshas.

The Ayurvedic Clock

You know the saying "timing is everything"? That's absolutely true not only in life, but also in Ayurveda. For instance, no matter how healthy a meal you prepare for yourself, if you're eating it late at night, you may actually be doing your body more harm than good. At night, your body's purificatory channels are in full gear, helping to rid your system of toxins and preparing a clean slate for the next day. Eating a heavy meal close to your bedtime bogs those channels down, leaving you feeling groggy and heavy (and possibly suffering from acid stomach) the next day. Here's where the Ayurvedic clock comes in, and why it's so important.

In the Western world, we tend to see the day divided into two 12-hour cycles of night and day. But according to Ayurveda, there are actually six daily cycles of four hours each that correspond to the doshas. In other words, there's a Kapha time of day, a Pitta time of day, a Kapha time of night, and so on. As you'd expect, Kapha qualities tend to be livelier during Kapha time, just as Pitta qualities are stronger during Pitta time and Vata qualities are stronger during Vata time.

As you read about these cycles, you'll gain some understanding about why your energy tends to ebb and flow throughout the day and night. Simply put: doshas rule the day! And as you learn about the Ayurvedic clock, you'll gain tips for how to better attune yourself with nature's rhythms all day long.

Daytime Kapha Cycle | 6:00 a.m. to 10:00 a.m. | Get Moving!

The daily cycle begins in the early morning with Kapha dosha. Because Kapha dosha is associated with earth and water elements, most people tend to feel a bit of heaviness and sluggishness at this time. If you're a Kapha-dominant person, this influence will be amplified!

The 6:00 a.m. to 10:00 a.m. window is an effective time to stretch your body, do some light yoga, go for a morning walk, or engage in light exercise to get your blood circulating. When the weather is warmer, get out and walk in the sunshine if possible. Not only does it make you feel fresh and invigorated, but it also elevates your mood.

Researchers from Northwestern University found that being outside in the morning light helps boost your metabolism for the entire day. Moreover, according to the Mayo Clinic, walking is recommended to help trim your waistline, strengthen bones and muscles, improve mood, and help with conditions like high blood pressure and type 2 diabetes.

Daytime Pitta Cycle | 10:00 a.m. to 2:00 p.m. | Focus and Eat Your Largest Meal

As the day progresses, the sun climbs higher in the sky and we move into the Pitta daytime cycle. At noon, when the sun is at its peak, your digestive fire is at its strongest as well. This is why Ayurveda recommends eating your largest meal of the day then, to ensure optimal absorption and assimilation.

Because Pitta dosha is associated with the element of fire, you may also notice that you feel particularly energetic during this time frame. However, it's not a great time to engage in physical exertion and exercise. The abundance of heat in your body and the environment at this time may lead to overheating, especially if you've skipped lunch to go for a run under the hot sun.

Pitta's daytime cycle (before and after lunch) is an excellent time for focus and learning—an ancient Ayurvedic principle that modern science now verifies. The general consensus among researchers is that the midday is the best time to learn new things and to study. In fact, a 2017 British study found that students who start school at 10 a.m. (rather than 7:30 or 8:00 a.m.) tend to learn better and more easily. As a parent, I find this fascinating! Getting kids to school during sluggish Kapha time (6 a.m. to 10 a.m.) can make mornings challenging for the whole family—never mind the fact that Kapha time is not conducive to proper learning.

Daytime Vata Cycle: 2:00 p.m. to 6:00 p.m. | Calm the Mind, Be Creative

From 2:00 p.m. to 6:00 p.m., we move into the Vata cycle. Vata dosha being associated with air and space, this is a good time for creative thinking and problem solving. It's also an excellent time to meditate and regroup, because the etheric energy in the environment is high.

If you're feeling grounded and balanced, you might notice some light, clear, expansive qualities of mental alertness during Vata's daytime cycle. If not, your mind might be all over the place and a little unsettled or scattered and unable to focus (afternoon lull, anyone?).

Some workplace environments now have rooms for meditation and yoga (that certainly wasn't the case when I was younger!), but even just a 5-minute pranayama breathing technique and a high-protein, low-carb snack with some herbal tea can help calm an overactive or fatigued mind.

Nighttime Kapha Cycle: 6:00 p.m. to 10:00 p.m. | Light Dinner, Early Bedtime

From 6:00 p.m. through 10:00 p.m., we move from the afternoon into the darker hours of the early evening—the nighttime Kapha cycle. At this time, you'll begin to notice Kapha's heavy, sluggish qualities once again. This Kapha time is why you might naturally feel the desire to unwind from your day and enjoy a light dinner, ideally several hours before bedtime.

Eat a lighter meal at dinnertime since your digestion will be slower. A heavier meal could result in disturbed sleep due to undigested food sitting in the stomach. Eating a heavy meal can also cause you to wake up feeling dull the next day.

Many people eat a lot at night, especially North Americans who are accustomed to eating a large dinner. This runs entirely counter to Ayurvedic principles. Some people graze throughout the evening while watching TV and then wonder why they don't sleep well and often feel nauseous in the morning. Well, now you know the secret to feeling great in the morning: eating a light, nutritious dinner the night before. Eating to excess at nighttime is a leading cause of weight gain and accumulated excess Ama.

To catch the proverbial *angel train* and enjoy a deep, glorious slumber, get to bed before 10:00 p.m. when Kapha's evening cycle ends. Get to bed by 9:45 p.m. for optimal results.

Nighttime Pitta Cycle | 10:00 p.m. to 2:00 a.m. | Sleep, Repair, and Restore

Pitta's fiery energy comes into play again from 10:00 p.m. until 2:00 a.m. Because Pitta governs metabolism and transformation in the mind and body, this is the time to metabolize and process the day's intake and experiences. Support your body's systems by being in bed and resting during Pitta's evening cycle. Think of it as the time when your body's nightly housekeeping crew comes in; the workers can't do their job if you're still up and eating or engaged in activity!

Many people get a second wind at 10:00 p.m., but this is a false energy. You may feel like Superwoman or Superman and start working on projects after 10:00 p.m., but then you look at the clock and suddenly it's 1:00 or 2:00 a.m. Sound familiar? Then you jump into bed and stare at the ceiling and feel horrible the next day.

Here's my advice (drawing on millennia of wisdom from Ayurveda): don't be a night owl unless you have to work the nightshift. It can wreak havoc on your health.

Nighttime Vata Cycle | 2:00 a.m. to 6:00 a.m. | Arise Early and Meditate

As Pitta flows into Vata time, the dosha's airy, etheric qualities usher in a precious time for expansive thinking and receptivity. Unlike Vata's daytime cycle, this isn't a time to engage in creative pursuits; it's a time to enjoy those last, lighter hours of sleep before arising early (ideally just before 6:00 a.m.) and engaging in meditation.

Many people like to exercise during Vata time, especially 4:00 a.m. to 5:00 a.m., but it's not ideal. Exercising during this delicate, etheric time can leave you wound up and hyper all day. If you've slept a solid seven hours beforehand, you can start exercising at 5:00 a.m. or thereafter; if not, you may be running on nervous energy all day.

People who have a lot of Vata in their system often find themselves waking up with their thoughts racing between the hours of 2:00 a.m. and 4:00 a.m. The culprit is usually excess worry, stomach acidity, or other types of indigestion. Early-morning insomnia can also happen frequently if you're over age sixty (in the Vata phase of life). Wi-Fi and screen time can be another huge factor in sleeplessness, especially among younger generations who often spend evenings glued to their phones or iPads. The good news is that solid slumber is doable, no matter your doshic makeup, age, or stage in life.

A good sleep starts the night before. Take care to relax and unwind, shut down all electronic devices, and enjoy a warm bath or some boiled milk during Kapha's nighttime cycle. It works wonders. Most of my clients find they're able to sleep straight through for seven to eight hours once they follow Ayurveda's helpful dietary and lifestyle recommendations.

A Note about the Ayurvedic Clock

If you are at the end of one dosha cycle and moving into another, you will likely feel the influence of both. That's why people often get drowsy and heavy-lidded early in the evening during Kapha time (6:00 p.m. to 10:00 p.m.) but then suddenly spring to life again when the clock strikes 10:00 p.m. and Pitta's evening cycle begins! As I mentioned above, getting to bed before 10:00 p.m. is one of the best things you can do to ensure a good night's sleep—and an energetic, productive day ahead.

Dinacharya: The Ideal Daily Ayurvedic Routine

Now that you understand how the daily dosha cycles influence your physiology's functioning throughout the day, let's go a little deeper and discuss routine. In Sanskrit, the word *dinacharya* translates to "daily routine." The ancient Ayurvedic practice of dinacharya is, essentially, a set of guidelines to help you organize your daily activity around the cycles of nature.

The Ayurvedic clock lies at the heart of the daily dinacharya. Knowing which dosha is particularly lively at any given point of the day will help you plan your meals for optimal digestion, exercise for optimal benefits, bedtime for optimal sleep, and so on. As with everything in Ayurveda, the goal is to harness nature's energy for optimal mind-body wellness and functioning.

Beginner's Tip: Go Easy on Yourself

The daily Ayurvedic routine can seem like a lot at first! But don't be overwhelmed. Remember: baby steps are the key to success. Start out with a few of these recommendations and notice how they improve your day. The more you make healthier choices for yourself, the better you'll feel (which makes it so much easier to make the next healthy choice). Before you know it, you'll be a dinacharya dynamo!

Morning Routine

Arise Early. Ayurveda recommends waking up early before 6:00 a.m. (when vibrant, dynamic Vata energy transitions into more sluggish, heavy Kapha energy). Ideally, you've had a good sleep because you went to bed before 10:00 p.m. the night before (before Pitta's dynamic evening cycle kicks in!).

Clear the Channels. Most of us naturally rush to the bathroom to urinate when we first awaken, but it's also helpful to train your body to evacuate the bowels first thing in the morning—or in those first few waking hours. Drinking a bit of warm water can help, but first make sure to clean your mouth.

Clean Your Mouth. Digestion begins in the mouth. Therefore, it's important to have a clean, fresh mouth so you can taste your food well. Cleaning your mouth the Ayurvedic way goes beyond just brushing your teeth, like we do here in the West. After you brush your teeth as usual, do your *Tongue Scraping*, followed by your daily *Oil Pulling*.

Tongue Scraping: This gentle technique is an age-old practice that helps clean the tongue of impurities. If your tongue is covered with a white or yellow filmy coating (a sign of ama), you won't be able to taste or digest properly. Ayurveda recommends gently cleansing the tongue of impurities with a stainless-steel tongue scraper (available online) or a spoon to remove any impurities deposited by the digestive tract the night before.

After brushing your teeth, firmly grasp the tongue scraper with both hands. Then stick out your tongue and place the scraper at the back of your mouth. Gently, but firmly scrape your entire tongue, moving from back to front. Repeat this a few times until your tongue looks and feels clean. Rinse your tongue scraper with hot water after each use.

In recent years, modern science has begun to recognize the value of this ancient practice. The Cleveland Clinic recommends: "Cleaning your tongue keeps ... bad bacteria, as well as food debris and dead cells that may accumulate there, from causing trouble." Other benefits of tongue scraping include fresher breath and more sensitive taste buds.

Oil Pulling: Ayurvedic texts also recommend oil pulling, where oil is used to pull impurities out of your mouth. After gently scraping your tongue a few times in the morning, swish a bit of organic sesame oil around in your mouth for a minute before spitting it out.

This practice helps to strengthen the gums and further remove impurities. Promising studies validate this ancient Ayurvedic practice, suggesting that oil pulling can kill harmful bacteria, reduce bad breath, and improve gum health.

Stimulate Your Organs. Many of us are naturally thirsty in the morning. Drinking a cup of warm water with a bit of lemon juice can help to stimulate your digestive organs and flush out toxins from the night before. If you suffer from constipation, drinking warm water is an excellent way to encourage regular daily elimination.

Alternatively, you can drink a cup of warm water that's been sitting overnight in a copper cup. Not only does it taste great, but it also sparks your body's purificatory channels, reduces acidity, and pacifies Pitta dosha.

Do a Soothing Self-Massage. Start your day with self-love by doing *abhyanga*. Anoint your body with warm herbalized oil to balance your doshas, stimulate circulation, enhance muscle tone, calm your mind, enhance well-being, and promote longevity.

Abhyanga is one of the best things you can do to calm your nervous system and tone your body, inside and out. That's why it's one of the basics of Ayurveda. Abhyanga has multiple benefits for mind, body, and spirit. It balances all three doshas (especially Vata) and is tremendously helpful for those who suffer from insomnia and nervous tension.

The health benefits of traditional massage are well documented within the scientific community, but new studies specific to abhyanga suggest that the practice reduces stress, lowers blood pressure, and promotes relaxation.

For directions on doing abhyanga, see the abhyanga section in chapter 8 later in this book.

Stretch and Strengthen. To shake off that early-morning stiffness and tone your muscles, do some gentle yoga asana stretches. That way, when you sit down for your morning meditation, your limbs will feel limber, invigorated, and comfortable.

Asanas and Sun Salutations: Long before computers and endless hours of sitting in cubicles, Ayurveda recognized the importance of gentle movements and exercises to keep the body limber and the mind refreshed. This is yoga, the sister science to Ayurveda. The two disciplines were developed together and work beautifully in tandem.

The goal of Ayurveda is to keep your body and mind healthy so you can experience true wellness—and beyond, to higher states of consciousness. The goal of yoga is to bring *prana* (life force) into your body and to free up the pathways for a higher level of experience. Gentle yoga stretches and poses (*asanas*) are an integral part of Ayurveda, as are the more vigorous sun salutations (*surya namaskar*).

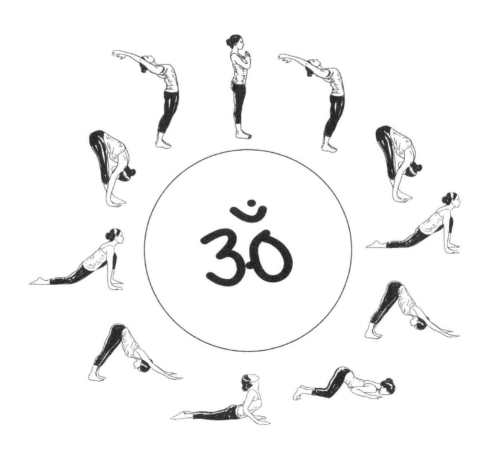

99

Get Your Prana Circulating. Prepare your body to sink into peaceful meditation by doing a few minutes of gentle *pranayama*. Breathing exercises help circulate prana throughout your body.

Pranayama (Ayurvedic breathing exercises): In our hectic, hurried world, we often forget to do one of the simplest things: breathe. Many people take only very shallow breaths. The practice of pranayama helps to draw breath, our life force, deep into the body in a nourishing, soothing way. The specific pranayama technique (alternate nostril breathing) I recommend in this book—and which is recommended by Maharishi Ayurveda—also helps to balance the left and right hemispheres of your brain.

Meditate for a Peaceful Mind. Set yourself up for a productive, balanced day by taking some time to meditate each morning. A calm, refreshed mind in the morning leads to more clarity throughout the day. See Chapter 1 for more on the Transcendental Meditation technique.

Eat a Healthy Breakfast. Eat a warm, nourishing breakfast, favoring foods in accord with your dosha type as covered in Chapter 2 on diet and digestion.

Get Moving. Kapha's daytime cycle (from 6:00 a.m. to 10:00 a.m.) is one of the best times for exercise. Take a short walk before work if you can. Better yet, ride your bike to the office to give your metabolism a boost for the rest of the day. Keep your dosha in mind when exercising.

Afternoon Routine

Make Lunch Your Biggest Meal. Your digestion is at its peak during Pitta time (10:00 a.m. to 2:00 p.m.), especially at noon when the sun is at its highest in the sky. For this reason, Ayurveda recommends making lunch the biggest meal of the day. Ideally, your lunch should be a delicious, warm meal that includes all six tastes (sweet, sour, salty, bitter, astringent, and pungent), but the main priority is to eat a balanced, satisfying meal rich in whole foods and fresh, cooked produce. Whatever you decide to make, eat according to your dosha.

Alternate between Rest and Activity. Ayurveda sees rest and activity as the keys to a balanced, successful life. Most of us will spend the majority of our weekday afternoons at work, running errands, and so on—in other words, being busy! Once things settle down a bit toward the end of the afternoon and early evening, find some time to unwind and meditate or do some calming stretches. Even just sitting quietly with a warm mug of tea can help you to decompress.

Evening Routine

Eat a Light Dinner. Around 6:00 or 7:00 p.m., eat a light dinner (think nourishing soups and stews rather than pizza, lasagna, or BBQ). Enjoy pleasant conversation in a quiet, TV-free environment. Be sure to leave several hours between dinner time and bedtime for optimal digestion. Remember: eating a big meal at nighttime can bog down your digestive system during the Pitta-dominant hours when your body needs to run through its nightly clean and repair cycle.

Take Time to Unwind. An hour or two before bed, unplug your devices and engage in some soothing activities to help you unwind from the day. Write in your journal. Take an easy stroll to see the sunset. Light some candles and chat with your loved ones. Draw a relaxing bath. The idea is to clear your mind before bed, so you don't take the day's worries with you to your pillow!

Get to Bed by 10:00 p.m. The angel train leaves at 10:00 p.m. when Pitta's nightly cycle kicks in. Whenever possible, get to bed around or before 10:00 p.m. to ensure the best night's sleep and a more wakeful, refreshed tomorrow.

Your Daily Ayurvedic Routine Checklist

Use this weekly checklist to keep track of how you're doing with your Ayurvedic routine! Remember, you don't have do everything on this list perfectly, or even every day—especially when you're just beginning to explore Ayurveda. The goal definitely is NOT to strain or cause yourself further stress by forcing any of these lifestyle changes. But the more of these things you do, the better you'll feel. Try it and see!

Your Daily Ayurvedic Routine Checklist

	Mon	Tues	Wed	Thu	Fri	Sat	Sun
Arise Early							
Evacuate Bowels and Bladder							
Tongue Scraping and Oil Pulling							

Drink Water							
Abhyanga							
Shower or Hot Bath							
Asanas							
Pranayama							
Meditation							
Healthy Breakfast							
Light Exercise							
Lunch: Biggest Meal at Noon							
Afternoon Rest and Reset							
Light Evening Meal							
Relax and Unwind							
Bed by 10:00 p.m.							

NOTES: How did you do with your new Ayurvedic routine this week? How do you feel? Have you noticed any changes in health or energy?

_____

_____

_____

_____

_____

Note your experience in the bottom section of the chart. You can photocopy this chart to keep track over a longer period of time.

Living in Sync with the Seasons

In the last section, you learned how each of the three doshas (Vata, Pitta, and Kapha) influences times of day and night. In the same way, these elemental energies govern the seasons within us and without.

In the cold, dark days of winter, we tend to burrow indoors, surrounding ourselves with warmth and comfort. In the heat of summer, we flock outdoors and shed layers to bask in the sun. You can probably guess which of the three doshas governs the heat of summer (hint: fiery Pitta). In this section, we'll explore which seasons are governed by which doshas, and how you can live in harmony with them all, no matter your Ayurvedic mind-body type.

We'll also talk about the different seasons of human life, from infancy through the golden years. I'll offer helpful insights and practical suggestions for staying healthy and balanced at every stage of life.

Vata Season: November through February

During Vata season the climate is starting to get cold, dry, and windy unless you are in a climate that doesn't have four seasons. From the Ayurveda perspective, any climate that possess those attributes at any time in excess is Vata aggravating.

Some areas where you live may be moister, but dryness also comes from heat or air conditioning that you use inside your house to stay warm or cool. Use a humidifier in your house with a device that gauges the humidity level so you can maintain the humidity at about 50 percent. In basements you might use a de-humidifier.

A cold or even warm wind will increase Vata as winds fan Vata's already airy nature. Walking in the wind and being outside for long periods of time during a windstorm are top activities that disturb Vata dosha. In such cases, be sure to wear a hat or scarf around your head and neck.

In addition, being out in extremely cold temperatures or doing outdoor sports like skiing and snowboarding will exacerbate Vata qualities. Just sitting in a cold house with little heat can aggravate your Vata. Always be careful that no part of your body is cold for long periods of time whether you are inside or outside. When your head, neck, chest, kidney, or bladder are cold for long periods of time, you can get an infection.

When I lived in New Mexico, I once took my daughter out in a baby jogger for a run. I was deep along the trail and far away from home when the winds suddenly picked up and the temperature dramatically dropped. I found myself in a full-blown, turbulent windstorm. Being from the East Coast, I had never experienced anything like this in my life. I was caught completely off guard. It must have taken me an hour to get back home walking against that strong wind although I tried to go as fast as I could.

When I finally arrived home, I had violent, excruciating cramping in my legs. I felt so weak. The wind left me bereft of any moisture and dried me out down to my bare bones. Add more wind, and you add more dryness. Ayurveda texts say the wind can make you mentally imbalanced as well, which is a nice way of saying temporarily crazy and out of sorts. I drank hot tea, did an oil massage, and enjoyed a hot bath. The next day I felt better, but it took a few more days for me to fully recover.

Athletes who spend time training outdoors will have more Vata disturbance than others, since intense exercise causes more dryness especially when the climate is both cold and dry. The general Vata-pacifying recommendations can mitigate long-term problems with dry joints, pain, and emotional imbalance.

Vata Recommendations

Use Vata tea, Vata spice mixture, and Vata massage oil (available online at Mapi.com).

Eat warm nourishing foods.

Follow a regular routine.

Use oils such as ghee and olive oil for cooking (people who use coconut oil in excess during colder seasons will find it impossible to get warm no matter how many layers they wear and how high the heat is).

Pitta Season: Summer, or July through October

Pitta dosha is extremely sensitive to heat and warmer climates. You may notice in the summer that people get more impatient and angrier than in other seasons. This is because people spend more time in the heat. If someone works in construction and is out in the sun all day working in high temperatures, this can cause lots of problems over the long term. Hence, outdoor work is not a good idea for pure Pitta people, especially during the summer season.

The heat absorbed in the summer builds up. As a result, anger and impatience can carry over into the later fall and winter season if you don't get it under control. Being in air conditioning, while it's good to cool down, also dries you out. The fluctuations of going from the ice-cold air conditioning to outdoor heat is also taxing on the physiology and the mind as well. You may notice this when you go into an ice-cold store or restaurant in the summertime. It's really not necessary to keep it that cold. In Europe and other parts of the world they maintain a more sensible temperature indoors. Extreme cold causes digestive issues.

Also, sunscreen won't protect anyone from the intense effect of being in heat for sustained periods of time, although it helps with sunburn. Pitta dosha burns more easily than other doshas, so always be covered completely so you don't get skin damage or skin cancer. It's okay to get some sun exposure on less sensitive areas such as your arms or legs to increase natural vitamin D levels but avoid direct sun on your face and chest.

Pitta Recommendations

Coconut and rose water are the two most cooling foods to use.

Avoid hot foods. Favor fresh local vegetables and cooked grains.

Coconut oil massage is very cooling. Then take a cold shower.

When we lose water, we can dehydrate quickly. Drink coconut water to replace electrolytes, cooling rice milk, or Pitta tea cooled to room temperature. Also eat watermelon and other melons.

Kapha Season: March through June

Kapha season is moist and cold. Since Kapha issues are primarily in the head and chest region, common problems are allergies, bronchitis, colds, and sinus problems. Kapha types need more balance. The moister and colder the climate, the more difficult it is for someone to deal with these problems.

People with seasonal allergies often start sneezing at the first sign of spring. This can cause itching anywhere in the body, but especially the face and nose area as well as watery eyes. Many people are truly miserable. Anyone who follows a Kapha-pacifying diet (reducing sugar, hard cheeses, and fried foods) benefits tremendously.

My assistant suffered from allergies most of her life. She started following my advice and also taking a supplement called Aller-Defense (available from Mapi.com), which works wonders. Start the supplement a few months before the season and also do a *nasya* twice a day with nose oil to keep your nasal passages clear of pollutants and pollen, which are the main causes of severe allergic reactions in the spring. Nasya is so basic (described in Appendix II, Sinus Problems), but it works.

I once had a consultation with a man who was constantly sick but unwilling to change his diet, lifestyle, or other activities. Initially, he came to me open to more natural relief, but when it comes down to it, he didn't really want to make any changes. Months later, he was still resisting change and feeling lousy. It was frustrating for both of us.

Usually, a Kapha individual is dragged to a consultation by a spouse who is Pitta dosha. Remember Pittas are driven, disciplined, and more open to change unlike their Kapha spouses. That's tough on me as a wellness consultant because I can't really help them. To help them, I need patient compliance, and I can't even get that with my husband sometimes. He is driven and highly focused when it comes to work, but diet and lifestyle not so much. Fortunately, he has well balanced doshas and emotions for the most part and had a good daily routine when we met, but he can't handle the great lengths one needs to go to for good health. Luckily, he has me to help.

No one heals you. You are healing yourself. For best results, though, I need compliance from those I work with. Kapha types are the most difficult to get to follow a plan, but once they do commit, the plan can be successful. Some people would prefer the quick fix from over-the-counter drugs compared to putting a few drops of oil in their nose, popping some herbal tablets, and easing up on heavy foods. These heavy foods, particularly hard cheeses and meats, cause the problems I mentioned above, but can also lead to diabetes, heart disease, and even cancer.

Since all disease begins in the gut and Kaphas already have a weak digestion system, heavy Kapha-increasing foods can clog the channels. The problem is Kaphas have such a strong constitution that symptoms don't appear sometimes until the health issue is more advanced. One notices Vata and Pitta issues more quickly. Plus, Vata and Pitta types can recover more quickly.

When Kapha problems arise, they can also bring lethargy, low mood, and weight gain. Kaphas, when they are imbalanced, can easily get depressed; especially when they get sick, they definitely reach a low mood. Fortunately, low moods can be managed with some dietary and lifestyle changes.

Spring is the best time of the year for everyone to detox. As the weather gets warmer, it can loosen the mucus, phlegm, and ama that is abundant in Kapha types and in individuals with a Kapha imbalance. I recommend a light Kapha-pacifying diet for everyone in the spring since everyone will benefit from clearing out the accumulated ama during this time.

Although I'm Pitta-Vata, I have suffered from sinus issues my whole life. Ayurveda has been a huge help in alleviating the issues. You may have family members, co-workers or friends who are always sniffling, sneezing, or blowing their nose. Kapha issues are always more chronic than Pitta- and Vata-related health issues. Those can come and go more quickly but treating Kapha-related health issues takes time as they tend to linger.

While spring is not necessarily cold, it can be moist. The rainy season can create a major disruption for Kapha. Kapha types thrive best in the summer since they are often cold and usually love the heat unless they are mixed with some Pitta.

I've spent a lot of time in California and although it can be drier, it is not as warm as one would think. In the spring, the evenings can get down to forty degrees and feel colder if you have been basking in the sun all day and are not prepared with extra clothing. The California climate would be ideal for Kapha types, though, because it is much less cold than the East Coast, and the humidity is not that high.

Kapha Recommendations

Drink warm drinks and eat warming herbs.

Eat lighter foods. Eat less. Limit salt intake.

Avoid sweetness and cold.

Season foods with cinnamon, fresh or dried ginger, coriander, and black pepper.

Laugh, play, and have fun. Dance, sing, and move more.

The Stages of Life

The different phases of our lives all have a corresponding dosha. Knowing these stages of life—infancy, childhood, adolescence, early adult, midlife, and maturity—will help you navigate through the years.

The Kapha Years: Infancy to about 30 Years Old

During the Kapha years, infancy through about 30 years old, people tend to have more colds, coughs, bronchitis, and throat issues such as sore throats and swollen tonsils. This is why some children always seem to have a runny nose or a cough, especially in the spring and winter. Many children have to have their tonsils removed or are always struggling to reduce tonsil swelling.

Over the Kapha time span, a healthy baby, child, teenager and/or young adult will have an abundance of ojas. Of course, a person with a Kapha constitution will have more ojas than Pitta and Vata types. Nevertheless, the Kapha time of life supports in everyone smoother, more unctuous skin, a strong mind, and good physical energy. However, the reason why children and young people suffer especially from the common cold and Kapha-related health issues is due to them being in this time of life. There can be both positive and negative aspects depending on how balanced they are.

When we think of young people, we admire them for their stamina and relatively strong immune systems. They have not lived enough years on this earth to accumulate toxins or ama as older people have. However, I find more and more children, teenagers, and college students have stress-related health problems. Since these are the formative years, I think it's wise for parents to do whatever they can to support their children's development and protect them from damaging their mind (brain cells) and their body.

If you explain to children and teenagers what's at stake and start early, you can help them make better choices. Sit down with them and review the fact that poor dietary and lifestyle choices such as eating excess sugar or fried foods as well as excess drinking, drugs, stress, and lack of sleep can cause them to lose brain cells and possibly lead to auto-immune disorders, mononucleosis, and other ails. Even if your child or teenager seems to be healthy and fine, bad choices can catch up with them later.

A great place to start: Eat healthier yourself. Cook healthier meals. Don't have tempting foods in the house. In addition, have a family discussion about health and offer knowledge and support to all members of your family, not just your children.

My daughter, now thirty-three, is hearing health ideas that I may have told her over the years. Earlier, she would just have rolled her eyes at me. Now, even her friends have studied Ayurveda and she's reading advice from holistic doctors who are saying the same things I told her years ago. So, don't give in no matter how much resistance you face. Be a role model and, chances are, they will eventually follow.

A friend from grade school would have fruits and healthy options with her when we would get together for events. I was there with my Twinkies or three-pack Hostess cupcakes, which I genuinely loved at the time. She preferred more fruit and rarely ate packaged cakes. My mouth would water for the fruit because it looked delicious.

I had another friend who was vegetarian, but her parents were not. She demanded salads and vegetable which I'm sure helped her later in life. This was over fifty years ago when the U.S. was not yet health-conscious, and vegetarians were not commonplace as they are now.

My daughter loved vegetables and fruits at a young age, because that's all I gave her. Our pantry was not laden with sugar and processed food, so her appetite for healthy foods developed. Of course, she did relish the thought of visiting her friends who had the best junk food in town and binging from time to time. But she began to notice the negative effect after eating these bad foods.

Poor diet and stress in children can cause anxiety, ADD and ADHD, depression, learning and behavioral problems, and more. Studies in schools show that when processed food is taken out and replaced with fresh healthy meals, these health issues improve.

The Pitta Years: 30-60 Years Old

In midlife, from thirty to sixty, you will likely have Pitta health issues such as headaches, ulcers, stomach acidity, acid reflux, heart attacks, high blood pressure, and stroke. You might also be afflicted with Pitta emotions such as anger, irritability, impatience, OCD (obsessive-compulsive disorder), perfectionism, and being critical of others.

On a more positive note, during the Pitta time of life, people will generally have more energy and dynamism, particularly those with Pitta constitution. During the Kapha time of life, young people need to sleep more and it's hard to get kids going. That's why parents wonder why their 25-year-olds can sleep ten hours a night if given the chance. This starts to change when people enter the Pitta time of life. Certainly, between ages forty and sixty, people start to need less sleep (but make sure it's at least seven hours).

In the early phase of the Pitta stage of life, when we shed Kapha's influence, emotions can become stronger. The perfectionism of Pittas can start to take hold as well. If perfectionism might become an issue, you will see it early on. As a parent, take notice. Pittas can be so hard on themselves—trying to be the best and perfect to a fault. They might start having problems sleeping and develop some anxiety. Their competitive nature wants to succeed at any cost. If you are alert, you might notice an imbalance that needs to be addressed.

Some people don't get truly motivated in their thirties, so they don't finally grow up until they get a secure, well-paying job, or the hobby they love finally turns into a paying profession. It could be that since the brain is not fully developed until around twenty-five, some young people take more time to figure out what they want to do in their lives.

Either way the brain is more fully developed at thirty, so a healthy person will certainly make better choices in all areas of their life. That's why the first phase of life (Kapha) is crucial to what happens over the next thirty years during Pitta time. It's like building a house. Either you start out with a good foundation, or you have to work on many repairs over time. My motto, "pay now or pay later," applies here. It's a good time to speak to your children about what's important, even until you are blue in the face.

Pitta is the time of transformation. Pitta's fire element is responsible for fueling many of life's major decisions and forming who you become as a person. Mental imbalances can develop at this time if the foundation is weak. I feel sad when I see people struggle their whole life with issues that could have been eliminated with a few effective prevention tools.

As far as the full development of the brain, every young adult will complete this at a different time, so it's hard to know exactly where someone is on that spectrum. But a true Pitta type at any age will be busy all the time working on something. They rarely sit idle. If someone has lacked motivation before thirty and still does during the Pitta years, then either Pitta is out of balance or that person truly has more Vata and Kapha in their constitution (so they lack the drive of a true Pitta type).

We as human beings and especially as parents need to accept and respect the different dosha types and their need to develop at their own pace. Drive and ambition can be overrated. As the saying goes, "Slow and steady wins the race."

The advantage of Kapha types is their tendency during the Pitta time of life to stay with a steady job. They don't get as easily bored with mindless, repetitive work like their Pitta counterparts. They can sit at their desks, do their work, and rarely butt heads with colleagues.

On the other hand, Pittas can get restless if they are unfulfilled in a job. They may also get impatient, yell at their bosses or co-workers, and risk getting fired. Pitta types are opiniated and critical. They constantly stir the pot. They resent employees who they feel are not pulling their weight or working as hard as they are. Pitta types need to understand that not everyone is inclined to work as hard as they do.

I wished someone had told me that when I was young. I had to figure it out later in life when I looked back and saw what a menace I had been in the workplace. I thought I was fighting for justice, even for other colleagues, but my efforts always left a lot of hard feelings on many levels, especially before I learned TM.

My mom can attest to the fact that the fight is in our DNA. She blames my dad's side (the Italians). They can be outspoken, and they always fight for justice. While this behavior is noble, it's not what you do but how you do it. I have learned to tone it down a bit by thinking before I speak. This is the biggest lesson for pure Pitta types during this period: do not overact in an impulsive way and upset people.

The Pitta phase of life is seen in greater dynamism in one's activities. Typically, any negative Kapha tendencies, such as sluggishness and lethargy of the mind and body, start to recede and Pitta's natural energy, vitality, and focus can be more influential. Pure Pitta types can often start out with a bang at age twenty or so, overflowing with ambition and intense focus. Other doshas with less Pitta qualities can at least gain more of these benefits during the Pitta time of life and take advantage of the new-found energy that might not be part of their inherent nature, or prakriti.

The Vata Years: 60 and Over

During the mature phase of life, from age sixty onward, Vata influence grows. You will likely have more Vata-related physical imbalances such as dryness, constipation, irritable bowel syndrome (IBS), colitis, diverticulitis, loss of balance, weak knees or hips, bone loss, dementia, Alzheimer's disease, Parkinson's disease, fibromyalgia, diabetes, and heart issues. You can also develop emotional imbalances such as anxiety, worrying over nothing, memory loss, focus problems, depression, or sleep issues.

Even though many people are quite healthy at age sixty or over and may feel like they are twenty, they soon realize they need to take better care of themselves. This feeling can start to happen around forty or fifty for those who are overworked or stressed out.

Sometimes, people who retire at age fifty or sixty find that their health declines based on how they took care of themselves over the prior decades. Way too many top professionals have had to leave high paying jobs due to health issues that doctors could not resolve. Their energy levels plummeted, and they struggled to regain their health using conventional medicine alone. Fortunately, they had the time to seek out more natural methods and have worked with me to restore their health.

When you are younger and don't take care of yourself, there is enough reserve ojas so you may get by for a while feeling good. However, during the Vata years, your body and your mind start to dry out more. Ojas is declining, so the goal is to do whatever you can to protect yourself from accumulating toxins or losing ojas too quickly.

Many people over sixty are in tip-top shape. You can see it by their demeanor and in the vibrancy of their speech and gait. They have taken care of themselves. Their rewards are fewer doctor visits and a better quality of life. They are mentally alert and physically capable well into their nineties. A person should be able to live until well over the age of one hundred and still be able to drive and care for themselves.

With digestion and the microbiome, Vata types can have more irregular digestion, and issues can emerge that you need to be careful about. A pure Vata type moving into the Vata time of life needs to be more alert to imbalances. They may have a hard time keeping a healthy weight, they can become too thin (which is not good either), and they also can have more aches and pains. During this Vata time of life, don't wear yourself out mentally or physically. Follow a Vata-balancing diet and routine to keep yourself healthy.

Worrying can become one of the main emotions at this time, and some aging individuals have trouble shaking the experience of worrying over nothing. It's a terrible state for anyone to be in at any time. But as you age, needless worry can zap your joy in life.

When a predominately Pitta type moves into the Vata time of life, the air quality of Vata can blow fiercely through the Pitta's body and cause an existing steady fire to become an inferno. Observe your emotions and those of your loved ones to spot something like this happening.

Often, we equate this change with the stereotypical grumpy person. Most families have one such relative, and you might be grumpy yourself. One pattern in many Pitta people is that if they have been impatient and irritable throughout their lives, it only gets worse as they get older. However, I've taken many impossible Pitta types, including myself, and calmed them down, making them less likely to fly off the handle. Often, taking a vacation and getting out in nature will help. Slowing down will also help keep all doshas in check.

Kapha dosha people moving into the Vata time of life have their own troubles. While they may have more Kapha and possibly some extra ojas on hand, often they have not addressed some longstanding health issues. They are slow-moving and slow to make changes. They have a tendency toward complacency and lack of exercise. They can have type-2 diabetes and Kapha-related problems of colds and congestion. Since both Vata and Kapha doshas are cold, they tend to be colder more of the time, which is why so many pure Vatas and Kaphas flee to warmer climates at the onset of the Vata stage of life. They suddenly find cold to be intolerable.

All doshas find that, during Vata times, creativity can increase. They also feel an inclination towards hobbies and other pursuits for change and stimulation.

If you've raised children and they have moved out of the house, the Vata period can free up more personal time for yourself. This is the life stage to go within and, if inclined, to get in touch with your spiritual self.

Fortunately, the senior years are not what they once were. People are not retiring at age fifty anymore. Many people stay with their careers much longer and then, in retirement, find a way to give back to society by volunteering and helping people. Transitioning to another realm can be scary for some, but if you embrace your spirituality, then you can embrace this third chapter of your life with grace and love for yourself and others.

Chapter 6: Maharishi Vastu Architecture

What is Maharishi Vastu Architecture?

Vastu Architecture has been practiced in India since 6000 BC, but as with most knowledge, diluted forms emerged over time and were not consistent with the traditional Vedic texts. Maharishi systematically worked with a team of Vedic scholars to revive and restore Vastu Architecture in its purest form.

One may take any type of standard architecture and incorporate Vastu principles. Its key elements are based on the impact of the sun and our relationship to the North Pole, South Pole, and equator. This means when you are deciding to build or live in a house, you would have a design that supports your emotional and physical well-being, livelihood, and spiritual life. By living in a dwelling using Vastu principles, your home will properly align your individual intelligence with all the intelligence in the universe.

Maharishi used the term *natural law* to describe how all aspects of life need to be in harmony with laws that exist on earth and in the cosmos (extending to the planets, sun, moon, and stars).

We tend to assume that the cosmos is separate from us; however, research and experience tells us that we are not separate. The laws have an influence and purpose in our lives.

"Because the individual life is cosmic, everything about individual life should be in full harmony with Cosmic Life. Maharishi Vedic™ architecture gives dimensions, formulas, and orientations to the buildings that will provide cosmic harmony and support to the individual for his peace, prosperity, and good health—daily life in accord with Natural Law, daily life in the evolutionary direction."
— Maharishi Mahesh Yogi

Proper Orientation of Your Home or Building

One of the most important features of Maharishi Vastu Architecture is that the structure where you live or work should faces east. This orientation will bring the best influence to increase the quality of life for the occupants, including greater success and happiness.

East-facing dwellings create the most success because the sun's influence is greatest and most nourishing first thing in the morning. For this reason, it is important that there isn't any delay in the sunrise reaching your home. As soon as the sun rises, its rays should reflect the front of your house. Since earlier morning hours are considered most supportive, it's best to avoid having any large buildings, mountains, or other structures obstruct the sun's rays.

North-facing dwellings are the second-best option for your home, but west-facing and south-facing are considered inauspicious. The building should not be more than a few degrees north of east, and it is unfavorable for the building to be south of east.

Always check with a certified Maharishi Vastu expert before buying or renting an apartment or home. Of course, it is difficult to conform apartments and condos because there may be multiple building entrances. If necessary, however, there are sometimes ways to adapt an apartment or condo to Vastu principles. Many Vastu experts provide rectification to improve the Vastu influence if you are unable to move.

Buildings with east or north entrances can promote greater success, happiness, spirituality, health, and fulfilling relationships. Improperly oriented houses can bring problems such as poor health, lack of success, relationship difficulties, and unhappiness.

Scientific research validates that the human brain is affected by the direction you are facing. East seems to be optimal for high brain wave coherence and clearer thinking. Whenever possible, face east while you study or work, either at home or in an office. You should also have your head facing east or south when you sleep. Facing north or west are not favorable and should be avoided.

About 75 percent of all buildings have inauspicious entrances. It's no wonder there are so many problems in the world. Such improper planning and construction should be corrected in order to improve our lives.

Real estate agents who work with people from Asia say that many are aware of the importance of proper entrances, so they ask the agents for east-facing or north-facing homes. I did the same with my realtor when looking for a home in the Chicago suburbs. Meeting all requirements listed in this chapter was not an easy feat, but I felt it was well worth it to ensure my family's health.

Placement of Rooms

Maharishi Vastu Architecture designs the placement of rooms as they relate to the sun moving around the house throughout the day. As the sun moves, its influence changes. As noted earlier, the east sun on the house brings energy and vitality to start the day.

The southeast corner of the house is ideal for the kitchen. The fire of the sun can stimulate agni, our digestion. Eating and cooking in the southeast corner stimulates digestion and ensures better health.

The northeast is for meditation because we do not want the stimulation from the southern influence as with digestion. Now we want a more inward influence of transcending and that can happen more easily with a room on the northeast corner. All traditional Vastu homes opt for the meditation room to be in that area. This room can be either on the first or second floor.

The owner of the house should sleep in the southwest. Guests and other family members can also sleep in the southwest or southeast.

The living room can be on the west side or in the center of the house.

Maharishi Vedic Architecture and Bau Biology

When Maharishi revived the principle of Vedic architecture, he incorporated many of the principles of Bau Biology. Both Maharishi Vedic Architecture and Bau Biology believe our modern lifestyle is the cause of many health issues Maharishi called *sick building syndrome*.

Some of the most important Maharishi Vedic Architecture principles for promoting better health include the following:

☐ Do not use toxic chemicals in furniture and building materials.

☐ Do not use building materials that don't breathe well and thus, can create mold.

☐ Lower radon levels.

☐ Lower magnetic and electric fields.

☐ Lower radio frequency.

1. Avoid toxic chemicals in your furniture and building materials.

The modern era ushered in the use of chemicals to manufacture household cleaning products, laundry detergent, paints, adhesives, deodorants, perfumes, air freshener, and furniture.

Homes and offices have become toxic in many areas. As a result, they are making people sick. Many of these toxins are barely detectable by sight, smell, or touch. Of course, if you see black mold in your home or you walk into a house and smell a musty odor, there could be a serious problem. Without an obvious smell, many people are not necessarily aware when there is an issue.

Common signs like allergies, respiratory problems, and other health issues can be related to building issues. Sadly, I have many clients who are sensitive to chemicals and other airborne irritants. They can't be in homes or buildings, for example, where there are heavy perfumes, mold, strong-smelling cleaning solutions, cats, dust, or pollen. Some clients are also sensitive to chemicals used on lawns and crops.

Sensitive clients often organize their life around this challenge. They avoid places which have indoor pollutants they can't tolerate. They also are careful outside where people might have used toxic chemicals on lawns or gardens at home, schools, or businesses. Those beautiful green lawns that look almost fake probably have terrible chemicals on them. For people with sensitivities, in the long run, needing to avoid chemicals in a polluted world is actually a net gain.

On the surface, you may not be bothered by any negative effects from chemicals, but then one day you develop headaches, respiratory problems, brain fog, autoimmune disorders, multiple sclerosis, fibromyalgia, tremors, or a host of other potential health issues. Such exposure has destroyed lives when people had to quit their jobs to focus on regaining their health.

Fortunately, worldwide awareness of environmental toxicity has become more prevalent, so we are beginning to correct the mishaps that the chemical era has wrought. Companies were forced to remove or reduce formaldehyde and other nasty chemicals from products. California led the way with stringent codes on what they allow and don't allow in products. In fact, when products arrive from China, they are required to have holes in the packaging on the inside of the box so the product can off-gas on the ship; otherwise, without the off-gassing during the shipping, they might not meet California standards.

Sadly, formaldehyde is used in baby cribs, which can have devastating health consequences for a newborn and may explain why mysterious health issues occur among babies and children. Formaldehyde is also used in the glue on new hardwood floors. This glue can affect dogs who sleep on the floors with their noses next to formaldehyde-glued planks. Children who crawl on these floors can also be affected in debilitating ways.

Over time, formaldehyde and other chemicals will off-gas, but sometimes not before tremendous damage has been done to the residents of the home. Babies and small children are often most affected, with exposure being more detrimental to their delicate lungs and other organs.

Some environmentalists believe formaldehyde does not off-gas completely. However, I had a test done after my new home was renovated and it showed no trace of toxic chemicals. To create the healthiest air possible, I used an excellent air purifier that kills mold, viruses, and other toxins.

At the end of this chapter, I recommend a few high-quality air purifiers and describe how to use them when renovating your house, moving into a new house, or bringing new furniture into your home.

Here's a tip: Unpack furniture and keep it out in the fresh air for a few days, or in your garage for a few weeks before you move it into your house.

Another tip: Allow fresh air to enter your home every day to continually move toxins out.

2. Use building materials that breathe and thus, don't create mold.

Although long-term exposure to mold will do the most harm, even short-term exposure can cause health issues. Mold exposure can cause respiratory problems, allergies, coughing, wheezing, and more serious illnesses such as cancer and autoimmune disorders.

Take any speck of black mold in your house seriously. Before moving into a house or apartment, have mold tests done. Just because you don't see or smell mold, doesn't mean it's not there. Testing is the key for detection, but also look around the house for moisture, water, and cracks. Any areas of the house where there are cracks (in caulking, wood floors, or tiles) are red flags that mold might be present. If there was a flood or excess water where the carpet got soaked, the pad underneath might never dry out and could create mold. Even a few weeks of dampness can cause problems.

I rarely recommend carpeting in homes, not only because of potential mold issues, but also because synthetic fiber carpets can off-gas and cause breathing problems. With wall-to-wall carpeting, it's often harder to see mold if it develops. Wool area rugs are generally fine, but synthetic fiber rugs are usually toxic. Also, some people can't handle wool in the bedroom; the only way you will know if you are sensitive to wool in your bedroom is to sleep in a room with a wool carpet for a night or two and see if any breathing complications come up.

It's best to have natural carpets and curtains in your home. Natural fibers, especially where you sleep, are part of the Vedic building requirements for healthy living.

Once you figure all this out and create a healthy home, you will feel the difference. It may take a few years for you to research and follow all the recommendations in this book. Being in a toxic environment for a few years is tolerable as long as you find a long-term solution. Most people's bodies can heal quickly once they are in a better environment.

In *Breathing Walls: A Biological Approach to Healthy Building Envelope Design and Construction*, George Swanson and Oram Miller explain the importance of using natural materials in a specific way so that you can achieve the right balance of moisture. While the book is mainly about building a house, it provides many tips you can use to renovate a room or improve your living space. The authors suggest appropriate resources for building materials as well.

Steps to take to fix a mold problem:

1. Do a mold test. Most experts know the most likely problem areas: under the kitchen sink, in the basement, and places where prior leaks have occurred.

2. Hire a mold remediation expert. If test results show that toxic mold is high, hire a mold remediation expert. If you've had a flood, some walls may need to be removed. I've been in houses that had multiple floods, and I can report firsthand that there is mold behind such walls. If you have an unused basement, leave walls open or remediate. Once remediation is completed, paint over the wood behind the walls with a mineral primer. This will inhibit mold from growing once you close off the wall.

3. Once remediation is complete, test for mold again. Use another company to test for mold a second time. If mold is present, make sure all affected walls are torn apart and all carpet or flooring is taken up. Start by tearing off part of a wall to verify that mold is present. Little by little, check all areas that might have been affected by mold.

For mold to grow, it needs moisture, darkness, and a food source. Once you clean out mold, follow the remediation guidelines in *Breathing Walls*. Once remediated, floors, ceilings, and walls can be painted with mineral paints that keep mold out. To be safe, call George Swanson, author of *Breathing Walls*, for a private consultation.

If you have a fan that can circulate air or an air-conditioning unit that brings in fresh air from the outside, you'll have fewer mold problems. Bringing fresh air into your home a few times a day, as Ayurveda recommends, will help you control most mold problems.

Pay attention to areas where water leaks often happen—in the bathroom, kitchen, laundry room, and wherever else there is a sink. Make sure the rim around the bottom of the toilet that meets the floor is not completely sealed; otherwise, if there is a leak, you will not know it's there. If it's unsealed and there is a leak, water will come out and then you can take care of the leak. Once a month, check the areas that could be a problem, so you don't have any surprises later. They can go unnoticed, especially if the leak is small.

3. Lower radon levels.

Radon is a gas produced by uranium and found in soil, rock, rivers, and oceans. Found in many homes throughout the U.S. and the world, high levels of radon can be dangerous. Since radon is the second-leading cause of lung cancer in the U.S., breathing radon over time increases your risk of lung cancer. In the U.S., the Environmental Protection Agency (EPA) estimates that 21,000 people die each year from radon-related lung cancer. Only smoking causes more lung cancer deaths.

Radon gas can enter a house through a broken foundation, crawl spaces, and sump pumps that are not tightly covered. Because of the known health risks, many states have mandated that radon levels be checked before selling a home. If a home doesn't meet EPA standards, the homeowner is required to pay for mitigation before a buyer takes ownership of the house.

Although the EPA requires that radon levels not exceed 3.9 picocuries per liter (pCi/L), it's better if the levels are as low as 1 or 2 pCi/L. To reduce radon gas, air out your house periodically. When you sleep, keep a window or two open.

Note: Radon levels can change naturally due to the settling of the house's foundation. This can occur due to fluctuations in temperature, changes in moisture or humidity, home renovations, or earth tremors that create cracks in a foundation.

This is what happened in the house I last bought. Testing revealed that the radon levels were over 40 pCi/L! That is dangerously high. The owner thought the test was wrong. No one had told him to check once every year or two.

As a result of the test, the owner was required to hire a company to find out where the radon was entering the house. When I toured the house, I had noticed that the sump pump was exposed. That's an easy fix. A professional radon mitigation company can install a unit in the home that sucks radon out into the open air. It does this quietly, so you won't even know the unit is there. The average cost for such a unit is around $1,000. In some cases, where two units are needed for a larger home or a home with extremely high levels, the cost may be around $2,750.

Instead of paying $200 for a professional radon inspection, you can buy a small digital radon detector that will show your radon levels. I use a Corentium Home detector (available from airthings.com). Owning a radon detector allows you to monitor your radon levels, especially if you have had high levels before.

If you choose to pay a radon inspector, they will come to your house and set up testing machines that test over a 48-hour period to gain an average. Use a licensed radon inspection company when buying a home so you can show the owner a professional estimate.

4. Lower magnetic and electric fields.

What are electromagnetic fields (EMFs)?

Electricity and magnetism are two related phenomena produced by the electromagnetic force. A moving electric charge generates a magnetic field. A magnetic field, in turn, induces electric charge movement, producing an electric current.

Where do we find these fields?

Electromagnetic fields (EMFs) supply electricity to power homes and businesses. EMFs are found in the electric wires in your home where you plug in your devices. You can also experience EMFs outside your home wherever you see power lines, high-tension wires, cell phone towers, and radio wave towers. EMFs include magnetic fields, radio waves, and electric fields.

Why are EMFs bad for your health?

To learn details of this complex subject, go to Oram Miller's website at CreateHealthyHomes.com. An expert Bau biologist, Miller has studied with the top people in the field.

"For over fifty years, the American Academy of Environmental Medicine has been studying and treating the effects of the environment on human health. In the last twenty years, our physicians began seeing patients who reported that electric power lines, televisions, and other electrical devices caused a wide variety of symptoms. By the mid-nineties, it became clear that patients were adversely affected by electromagnetic fields and becoming more electrically sensitive.

In the last five years with the advent of wireless devices, there has been a massive increase in radio frequency (RF) exposure from wireless devices as well as reports of hypersensitivity and diseases related to electromagnetic field and RF exposure. Multiple studies correlate RF exposure with diseases such as cancer, neurological disease, reproductive disorders, immune dysfunction, and electromagnetic hypersensitivity." — American Academy of Environmental Medicine

---

Magnetic Fields

Outside overhead or underground power lines: There are many reasons why two houses have the same number and size of power lines and yet one house has magnetic readings at normal levels and the other has high readings at extremely dangerous levels. One house might have a main electrical box on its property that supplies the whole block. Or the house might have underground pipes close to the power lines. Or sometimes a house might have higher magnetic readings due to interactions of smart meters around the house, including influences from smart meters outside neighboring homes. You can avoid some of these negative magnetic readings by having a lot size of at least one-half acre. The further away your home is from any negative influences, the more the intensity of magnetic fields drops.

High-tension wires: High-tension lines are large and long, with the largest ones being the most dangerous. While most high-tension lines are placed along major highways or railroad lines, sometimes they end up running along someone's backyard. If that is the case for your home, think about moving. You don't want your home closer than a few thousand feet, or about three or four blocks, to high-tension lines.

Don't rely on a distance measurement. Use a good meter. It's better to measure magnetic fields rather than guessing.

Magnetic fields can also result from sources within a home, such as electric breaker panels, motors, transformers, and smart meters (which are worse than older analog meters). Toxic magnetic fields can also happen when your home or office wiring are installed improperly, resulting in currents running on metal water pipes or not being grounded.

Radio Waves and Wireless Communications

Radio waves are all around us, generated by some of the following modern conveniences:

- ☐ Cell phones, cordless phones, and cell phone towers
- ☐ Microwave ovens
- ☐ Radios, TVs, and radio station towers
- ☐ Air traffic control and car navigation systems
- ☐ Remote-controlled toys
- ☐ Wi-Fi, mobile hotspots, home entertainment systems

As you can see from the above list, many items in our daily life use radio frequencies. Due to their prevalence in our lives, radio waves have been blamed for an increase in cancers. For instance, talking on a cell phone next to your ear has been blamed for brain fog, headaches, brain tumors, sleeplessness, and more. EMFs, especially Wi-Fi and radio frequencies, can amplify existing diseases by 200%.

While most doctors can't explain these connections, anyone affected by radio wave sensitivity finally makes the connection. What they are experiencing is *electrical hypersensitivity* (EHS) or *electromagnetic field intolerance syndrome* (EMF-IS).

When cell phone towers were first erected, most were put near highways rather than near people's homes. But later, as people became comfortable seeing the towers, things changed. Cell phone towers began to pop up in backyards, parks, schools, churches, and office parks.

Homeowners, churches, schools, and workplaces that adopt a cell phone tower are paid a monthly fee by mobile operators for the use of their land. If people knew the negative affect on their health, they would think twice about having cell phone towers right next to their homes. Now with 5G cell phone networks expanding, there could be a cell phone tower every five feet on your block.

Currently, 5G networks have not fully rolled out in all cities, suburbs, and states, but they will be ubiquitous very soon. Right now, most areas outside of major cities are currently running 4G with existing cell phone towers. However, because they are closer to our work and homes than they should be, the levels exceed what is acceptable for good health.

How can wireless 5G impact your health? With 5G radio waves being more intense than 4G, all cancers and other illnesses could develop more quickly and end up being more serious.

Dirty Electricity

Electric fields in the wires of your house can cause dirty electricity (spikes and surges of electromagnetic energy that travel along power lines and building wires). Once you reduce the magnetic and radio frequency fields, work on the electric fields surrounding your TVs and computers, dimmer switches, and compact light bulbs.

Because magnetic fields and radio frequencies can increase the negative effects of electrical fields, start with the magnetic and radio fields so you can see a realistic baseline. To minimize dirty electricity, buy inexpensive shielding or filters (available at RFReduce.com).

Maharishi Vedic Architecture and EMFs

One recommendation of Maharishi Vedic Architecture is to choose a home that does not have high levels of EMFs. Homes should not be built or located near harmful electromagnetic fields caused by high-tension power lines and cell towers. The typical power lines found on your property are generally safe since they are usually a distance away from your house—and harmful levels typically drop off as distance increases. However, with the introduction of smart meters, many people feel that EMF levels have increased to unsafe levels.

If you are building a Vastu home, an electrician can configure your home's wiring to ensure that electromagnetic fields are not propagated within your home. The electrician just needs to follow a design created by an EMF expert. Vastu guidelines consider electromagnetic fields so when a home is built following these guidelines, EMF levels should be safe for your health.

Vastu design also includes a switch in the bedroom that shuts off the electricity to reduce EMF fields while you sleep. To improve your health, minimize EMF field interference during sleep. When you work outside the home or in a large city, it's harder to control EMF fields, so it's important to reduce EMF fields in your bedroom. This EMF reduction allows your body to be fully restored during sleep.

Have you ever felt a sense of calm in a house when the electricity went out due to a storm? It might feel like a buzzing or vibration has stopped. This can happen when electrical currents stop running through your body. It's like the calm that comes over a person after returning home from a busy workday in the city. When you return home at night, you can really settle down from the buzz of the day.

Some people love big cities; they feel revved up and energized by urban living. But the same people often love getting away to the beach or to the country—not just for the quiet but also because the beach and the country have lower EMFs. Both the quiet and the lower EMFs help to restore a person's physiology.

If I were a city mayor, I would encourage homeowners to test their houses for EMFs and to configure their electric wires to protect their health.

5. Lower radio frequencies.

The closer you live to a cell phone tower, the higher the radio frequency becomes. With 5G cell networks, not only do they send out stronger signals, but also the towers are situated closer to homes and offices. EMF experts feel that the more 5G is implemented, the more humans will get sick. Trees, plants, and wildlife might also suffer.

While looking for a home in the Chicago suburbs, I measured 4G levels in many neighborhoods. I discovered that houses closest to cell phone towers always have the highest EMF readings. With 5G, these towers will become more ubiquitous and closer to homes. And, because 5G towers send out more powerful radio waves, they could easily affect your health. One doctor I know believes that Wi-Fi and other radio frequencies double your risk for any disease.

Mieke Jacobs had been relatively healthy while growing up. Shortly after arriving at Yale University, she started feeling more and more fatigue, which worsened when she moved to New York City after graduation. Eventually, because of her chronic fatigue, she returned to suburban Chicago. Her health improved after a while, but then she started having a different set of symptoms.

Only after many years of intense study did she determine that EMFs showed the strongest correlation with the ups and downs of her health. She finally figured out that her childhood home had been the only truly low-EMF place she had ever lived. Her health was much better there than in the college dorms, her New York city apartment, and the series of rentals she lived in after her childhood home was sold.

Although most people don't know much about the danger of EMFs, some people are working against the proliferation of 5G. They can already feel the danger of spreading such intense radio waves into more areas, especially residential neighborhoods.

Is there a connection between cell phone usage and brain cancer? As cell phone use increased, many brain surgeons reported seeing more brain cancers in teenagers and adults than ever before. Even singer Sheryl Crow noticed that her benign tumor was in the exact spot where she held her cell phone when talking.

Have you ever felt a burning or tingling on the side of your head after using your cell phone? Are you starting to forget where you left your car keys? Are you having more trouble remembering things? These are signs that you might be having health effects from using a cell phone or cordless phone.

The cell phone industry and governmental agencies, at least on this side of the Atlantic, claim that cell phones are safe, but some research indicates that might not be the case. Studies are being cherry-picked to hide the true health risks of cell phone use. Americans are not being told what Europeans have known for years: wireless communications can cause a host of medical problems.

These problems can include memory loss, brain fog, chronic fatigue, ADD, early-onset dementia, and cancer. Brain tumors and strokes among people in their twenties are on the rise. Young children who use cell phones have a five-fold increase in the rate of leukemia. Sadly, these health effects are cumulative.

Some studies show that humans are affected by two frequencies transmitted by wireless devices, including cell phones, cordless telephones, and Wi-Fi in routers and computers.

Each cell phone on the market has a Specific Absorption Rate (SAR)— and no cell phone can be sold if its SAR is beyond the level known to cause ill health. In Israel, manufacturers are required to post the SAR for each cell phone on display in a store, but in the U.S. that information is buried in the back of your cell phone manual.

SAR refers to the heating effect on cell proteins from the carrier wave, which is in the gigahertz (billions of cycles per second) range. But the SAR is not the problem. What worries scientists most is what is known as the low-frequency Information-Carrying Radio Wave (ICRW), which is the actual frequency that carries the voice data from the cell phone to the cell tower and back again.

The ICRW causes numerous health problems that are not currently being revealed by the industry—problems such as damage to the blood-brain barrier, formation of stress proteins and precancerous lesions, and loss of the ability of cells to communicate with each other.

This low-frequency ICRW is too weak to be transmitted by itself, so it is piggybacked onto a much faster heating frequency in the microwave range. The problem is we are exposed to both frequencies. And, sadly, health effects are mounting.

What Can You Do?

Wire Your Home

You can wire your home back to the way it was a decade ago with a landline and an ethernet cord. Do you know that all wireless technology requires wires somewhere? That means wireless isn't totally wireless. Ethernet offers a better connection for working at home. You can still use your cell phone when you are traveling but, at home, you can forward your text messages to your computer. Wiring your home and not using Wi-Fi can be a lot of effort, but it's a lot less effort than being sick.

Paint Your House

If you live close to a cell phone tower but love your home, paint your house with YShield High Frequency Shielding Paint (available online). This special paint has had great reviews for being effective in dramatically reducing radio frequencies. The paint is black, which isn't all that pretty, but you can cover it with regular paint of any color.

Keep Cell Phones at a Distance

When you must travel and use your cell phone, keep it at least six to ten inches from your body. Install a landline to use while you're at home. When you travel, use your cell phone on speaker mode rather than holding it up to your ear. You can also get an EMF blocker to reduce radio frequencies while you use your cell phone.

EMF Solutions

Here are some of the meters, filters, signal tamers, and other solutions to help you tamp down EMF fields, cellular fields, and radio waves.

EMF Trifield meter (Model TF2):
http://www.lessemf.com/combi.html#150-tf2

Bed Canopy—I recommend the Naturell but make sure to buy both the canopy and the floor mat:
https://slt.co/Products/BedCanopies/BedCanopySwissShieldNaturell.aspx and https://slt.co/Products/BedCanopies/BedCanopyFloorMat-Naturell.aspx.

Ethernet cable, Cat 6a, 7 or 8:
https://www.amazon.com/gp/product/B004NPL4YE,
https://www.amazon.com/gp/product/B00CJLEHPM, and
https://www.amazon.com/s?k=cat+8+ethernet

Wired keyboard and mouse for PC laptops: Check on Amazon.

Ethernet adapter for iPhones and iPads, Belkin Ethernet + Power Adapter with Lightning Connector:
https://www.amazon.com/gp/product/B07BMVW62P

Air Tube headset: https://www.smart-safe.com/collections/radiation-free-headsets/products/radiation-free-air-tube-headsets

Router guard: LessEMF.com sells a few different ones. Measure your router and ask which would fit best.

Signal Tamer: https://www.lessemf.com/computer.html#220

Wave Cage: https://www.lessemf.com/cellphon.html#755 and https://www.lessemf.com/cellphon.html#756

EMF SleepSafe circuit cutting switch: https://emfsleepsafe.com

DNA dirty electricity filters: http://rfreduce.com/mxdna3/

3-Prong shut off switches (so you don't have to plug and unplug your lamps all the time, just flip the switch): https://www.amazon.com/gp/product/B0113VTPSW/

USB ground cord (if your laptop doesn't have a 3-prong grounding plug): http://www.lessemf.com/computer.html#295-usb

EMF Research

5G EMF Hazards, click here for a free ninety-page PDF: https://peaceinspace.blogs.com/files/5g-emf-hazards--dr-martin-l.-pall--eu-emf2018-6-11us3.pdf

BioInitiative.org, Henry Lai's Research Summaries: https://bioinitiative.org/research-summaries

EMF Analysis: https://www.emfanalysis.com/research

EMF Research: https://www.emfresearch.com

EMF Wise: http://emfwise.com/science.php

Environmental Health Trust, Science and Policy Issues: https://ehtrust.org/science

Micro Wave News: https://www.microwavenews.com

Powerwatch Science Database:
https://www.powerwatch.org.uk/science/science-db.asp

Safer EMR: https://www.saferemr.com

Wi-Cancer Studies (Showing Health Effects from Wi-Fi Radio Frequency Radiation), click here for a free seventy-three-page PDF: http://www.wi-cancer.info/download.pdf

Air Purifiers and How to Use Them

Aran Air Purifier

The Aran unit smells like fresh air and is great for killing odors and purifying deeper toxins like formaldehyde that a HEPA filter can't handle. You can keep the Aran air purifier running continuously as long as the unit is not too large for the space. The team at Pure Air for Life can guide you on which unit to buy if you give them the dimensions of your house.

If you have new furniture or a room that has just been painted, close the doors, make the room as air tight as possible, and leave the unit running when no one is in the room. Doing this will remove the toxins at a faster rate. Air out the room when possible and run the unit again in an airtight room. You can read about how the Aran air purifiers work here: http://pureairforlife.biz/product-info.html.

HEPA Filters

HEPA filters do not smell like oxygen and will not make a room smell better. As long as it's running, however, a HEPA filter will kill almost anything in the air.

HEPA filters do a great job of capturing particles, but they don't filter out VOCs (volatile organic compounds). To remove formaldehyde and other VOCs, you need an air purifier with additional technology. Note: Air purifiers with activated carbon or granulated carbon are not as effective in removing VOCs as the Aran Air Purifiers.

Chapter 7: GMOs and Health

GMO (genetically modified) foods may not be good for your health. In this chapter, we will go into more detail about the potential harm from GMO foods and provide strategies to minimize exposure to these dangers.

GMO foods are controversial. Many people say that GMO foods have negative effects on people's health, while GMO proponents say they are safe to eat. To assess GMO effects, we'll cover compelling scientific evidence on the potential damage to people's health as well as anecdotal evidence that suggests real-life dangers to people's health. Finally, we'll suggest some steps you can take to mitigate this risk to your health.

Our main recommendation is simple: Favor an all organic diet to reduce the risk from GMO food. When people switch to an organic diet, they often notice significant improvements in their health.

What Are GMOs?

GMO stands for *genetically modified organism*. The term *GMO* can apply to both plants and animals. Genetically modified organisms are developed through manipulations in a laboratory, where genetic engineering alters the genetic material of an organism. Foods that have been genetically modified are not as natural as foods that are created from crossbreeding or plant breeding. Creating a new plant through cross-pollination leads to a more organic result than creating a new plant through genetic engineering.

The most common reasons food producers create GMO foods are to improve the resistance of the crop to herbicides (chemicals to kill unwanted weeds and plants) or to create an insecticide within the crop itself (an engineered part of the plant that kills unwanted insects trying to eat the crop).

GMO foods can be harmful to human health. Here are just a few of the reasons GMO foods can cause health problems:

☐ **Herbicide Residue**—Since GMO crops can be designed to be resistant to herbicides, larger quantities of herbicides can be sprayed on such crops. As a result, a larger residue of herbicide can remain on the crop when it is harvested, which can cause health issues for consumers.

☐ **Insecticide Damage**—Studies show that insecticides added to the crop through genetic engineering can cause damage to animals and humans who eat these crops. The damage can lead to immune system problems, tissue damage, and leaky gut.

☐ **Plant Modifications**—The process of manipulating the genes within the plants can introduce modifications to the composition of the plant that will cause harm to the consumer.

Major GMO Crops

GMO crops have become widespread in our food supply today because major GMO crops are key ingredients in many packaged foods. For example, 92 percent of field corn, 94 percent of soybeans, and 98 percent of cotton are grown from GMO seeds in the U.S., while 95 percent of Canadian-grown canola is from GMO seeds.

If you check the ingredients of processed foods in a grocery store, you will find at least one of these major crops listed in a majority of the items. Most likely, more than 50 percent of the processed food products you look at will have an ingredient derived from corn, soybeans, cottonseed, or canola. In other words, if you don't consciously try to avoid GMO foods, you are probably eating GMO foods in your daily diet.

Here is a partial list of some of the common food ingredients that are sourced from a GMO crop: vegetable oil, vegetable fat, margarine, soy lecithin, soy flour, soy protein, tofu, corn syrup, and cornstarch. Since these ingredients are found in so many other foods, always check the ingredients in processed foods you buy.

Minor GMO Crops

Other crops that have GMO versions available in stores today are apples, potatoes, papayas, lentils (from Canada), sugar beets, zucchini, and yellow summer squash. The percentage of these foods that are GMO is much less than with the major crops (with the exception of sugar beets, which are 95 percent GMO).

About 30 percent of the alfalfa grown in the U.S. is GMO. Since alfalfa is used to feed livestock, GMO ingredients can be passed on via meats or dairy products, including milk, butter, cheese, and yogurt. If a cow is feeding on GMO alfalfa, any dairy products from that cow are not considered organic.

Genetic engineering has also been used to create the bacteria that produce the artificial sweetener aspartame, known by such brand names as NutraSweet, Equal, and Canderel. Aspartame is widely used as an ingredient in foods. A 2018 study published in *Molecules* has shown that aspartame can have a toxic effect on gut bacteria.

Avoid sugar if it comes from sugar beets, since 95 percent are genetically modified. Instead, use sugar from 100 percent sugarcane, which, as of this writing, is not genetically altered.

Health Risks from GMO Foods

The debate about the health risks of GMO foods has been going on since the 1990s, when the first GMO foods were approved by the FDA and distributed. In spite of approval by the FDA, many scientists do not agree with allowing these foods to enter the general food supply. Their reservations are based on several scientific studies showing the harmful effects of these foods on both animal and human subjects.

Due to the growing number of studies documenting the health risks from GMO foods, more than sixty countries have enacted legislation to restrict or ban the production and sale of GMO foods.

The scientists who are concerned about the risks of GMO foods have argued that more long-term testing needs to be done before such foods are released to the public. Currently, few human tests have been conducted on GMO foods, which means we really don't know the full extent of potential damage from these foods. Especially concerning is that animal studies have demonstrated generational effects (negative effects that are passed down to future generations)—and yet regulatory bodies have thus far failed to require any long-term human studies. One difficulty is that human tests are typically not legal, so the only way to test GMO effects is to compare populations that are voluntarily eating GMO foods with populations that are voluntarily avoiding GMO foods.

The best tests exploring the dangers of GMO foods have been conducted on animals. If these foods are found to be dangerous to animals, there is a good chance they are also dangerous to humans.

Some potential risks that have appeared in research done so far (mostly animal studies and human cell studies done in labs) include:

- [ ] Increased risk of allergic reaction in both humans and mice to GMO foods

- [ ] Severe organ damage and hormonal disruption in rats in a long-term study using GMO corn

- [ ] Increased rates of large tumors and mortality in rats in a long-term study using GMO corn

- [ ] Increased precancerous cell growth in the digestive tract in rats in a study using GMO potatoes

- [ ] Increased stomach lesions (bleeding in the stomach) and mortality in rats in a short-term study using GMO tomatoes

- [ ] Increased toxicity in liver and kidney in a variety of animals in a group of studies using GMO corn, canola, and soy

- [ ] Enlarged lymph nodes, increased white blood cells, and decreased immunity in mice in a study using GMO triticale (a hybrid of wheat and rye)

- [ ] Decreased fertility in rats in a long-term study using GMO soybeans

- [ ] Increased sterility and reduced conception rates in pigs and cows in a study using GMO corn

- [ ] Increased rate of death of offspring in female rats in a study using GMO soybeans

- [ ] Increased liver inflammation in rats in a study using GMO canola

- [ ] Increased mortality rate in chickens in a study using GMO corn

□ Increased levels of insulin-like growth factor (IGF-1), a hormone considered to be a high risk factor for breast, prostate, colon, lung, and other cancers, in milk produced by cows treated with a genetically engineered bovine growth hormone (rbGH)

For more details on these studies, see "GMO Myths and Truths" (Earth Open Source, 2014) at https://livingnongmo.org/learn/resources.

Herbicides and Pesticides

When considering the health risks from GMO food, it is essential to include a discussion of the health risks from herbicides and pesticides. First, some GMO foods create an insecticide within the crop, and traces of that insecticide can appear in the animal or person consuming that crop. Second, when farmers are growing a GMO crop that is more resistant to herbicides, they use a larger quantity of herbicide on the crop, and traces of that herbicide will end up in the food supply.

What's important to understand is that pesticides and herbicides are dangerous to human health. They can be dangerous to the people who apply the herbicides and pesticides to the crop as well as to the people who eat food that has been sprayed.

Due to the growing number of studies about the dangers of herbicides, forty countries have either banned Roundup (the most popular herbicide used today) or are in various stages of banning or restricting its use. The list includes Canada, England, Germany, France, Australia, India, and Mexico.

Even though the United States is not on this list, the Centers for Disease Control and Prevention has recognized that more than 90 percent of the U.S. population have detectable amounts of pesticides in their blood and/or urine (https://www.cdc.gov/exposurereport).

Here are some findings related to the risk of herbicides and pesticides.

Pesticides added to the genetic code of the plant: For example, GMO corn has a pesticide called *Bt toxin* (bacillus thuringiensis) added to the plant via a genetic change. As a result, insects eating this crop die because their intestines break open. In addition, a study that fed such modified corn to rats reported that those rats experienced organ toxicity (*The Journal of American Science*, 2012).

Herbicides: The main herbicide used on crops is Monsanto's Roundup with an active ingredient called *glyphosate*. This herbicide is dangerous both to those who are spraying the herbicide and those who are eating crops that have been treated with it.

Glyphosate is the main active ingredient in Roundup, but other ingredients in Roundup (called *adjuvants*) are also toxic. These adjuvants make the toxicity of Roundup much more dangerous than glyphosate alone. In one study, the complete formulation of Roundup was found to be a thousand times more toxic to human cells than any individual ingredient (*BioMed Research International*, 2014).

Roundup is the most widely used weed killer in the world. In March 2015, the World Health Organization's International Agency for Research on Cancer (IARC) concluded that Roundup was "probably carcinogenic to humans." According to an IARC monograph, the cancer most directly associated with Roundup is non-Hodgkin lymphoma.

Thousands of lawsuits were filed between 2015 and 2020 against Monsanto (now Bayer) alleging that Roundup caused cancer in individuals working with the product. Finally, in 2020 Bayer agreed to pay approximately $11 billion to settle thousands of these lawsuits.

A report published in the *Journal of Hematology and Oncology (2019)* showed that a number of cancers can result from Roundup use, including colon cancer, liver cancer, pancreatic cancer, kidney cancer, melanoma, thyroid cancer, bone cancer, and breast cancer.

According to a 2007 study published in *Genetics and Molecular Biology*, researchers in Ecuador discovered a higher degree of DNA damage in the blood cells of workers using Roundup when compared to a control group. The study ruled out other possible causes, such as tobacco, alcohol, nonprescription drugs, and asbestos. The study also found other harmful effects from Roundup use: intestinal pain, vomiting, diarrhea, fever, heart palpitations, headaches, dizziness, numbness, and breathing difficulties.

Several other studies have shown harmful effects from Roundup use, including disruption of hormonal systems, negative impact on beneficial gut bacteria, developmental and reproductive toxicity, damage to DNA, cancer, and neurotoxicity.

Eating Food Sprayed with Roundup

In addition to the danger of working directly with Roundup, there is a risk when eating food sprayed with Roundup. Since GMO crops have been modified to be more resistant to Roundup, farmers often spray larger amounts on the crops. This heavy spraying can result in some herbicide residue remaining in or on the food itself.

An Iowa study, published in 2013 in *Food Chemistry*, found that GMO soy crops contain high residues of glyphosate and its breakdown product AMPA (aminomethylphosphonic acid), while non-GMO conventional and organic soybeans contained neither of these toxins.

GMO crops, engineered to be able to withstand the application of Roundup, have been found to absorb the glyphosate into their tissue. So, it's not just that there is some residue of the spray on the exterior of the plant, but the plant is also absorbing the glyphosate into its tissue. This means that consumers are eating the glyphosate directly when eating GMO foods. Technically, the plant absorbs some glyphosate and breaks the rest into a chemical called *aminomethylphosphonic acid*.

Both glyphosate and AMPA are toxic to humans. Laboratory studies reported in *Environmental Toxicology and Pharmacology* have shown that these two toxins can damage DNA in human cells.

A study published in 2012 in *Food and Chemical Toxicology* showed that rats fed GMO corn treated with Roundup suffered severe organ damage over a two-year period as well as increased rates of tumors and premature death. Most animal studies researching the damage caused by Roundup were done for only ninety days, and this longer study found that the significant damage did not appear until after ninety days. Existing studies are not meaningful if they do not capture long-term effects. As a result, it is misleading if a pro-GMO scientist says they have proven no damage from Roundup by citing a study that lasts only three months.

Animals and GMO Foods

Many farmers tell stories about animals refusing to eat GMO crops because they prefer more conventional crops. This is in-line with the expression, "Nature knows best." In *GMO 101: A Practical Guide*, chef Alain Braux reports the following:

- A Midwest farmer noticed that his pigs refused to eat GMO corn, but were more than happy to eat conventional corn feed.

- Farmers in Iowa offered their cows both GMO and conventional corn, but the cows would only eat the conventional corn.

- Farmers in Minnesota noticed that elk, deer, raccoons, and rats all avoided GMO grains.

- A farmer in Illinois noticed that migrating geese would eat only conventional soybeans and ignored the GMO soybeans.

GMO Crops and the Environment

Beside the health effect, GMO feeds and herbicides can also impact the environment and the economic health of farmers.

In terms of the environment, a study published in 2013 in *Insect Conservation and Diversity* revealed potential impacts from GMO farming. Carried out in the Midwest, this study discovered an 81 percent decline in the monarch butterfly population between 1999 and 2010. It also found a 58 percent decline in the milkweed population. Because milkweed is a prime source of food for the monarch butterfly, the researchers concluded that the increased planting of GMO herbicide-resistant maize and soybeans led to an increase in herbicide use which, in turn, killed off the milkweed plant which, in turn, resulted in the death of a large part of the monarch butterfly population. This finding illustrates the environmental cost of GMO foods: damage to what scientists call nontarget organisms, in this case, butterflies.

GMO farming itself can also negatively impact the environment. GMO crops often require more water, more chemical fertilizers, more herbicides, and more pesticides than conventional crops. The result is more chemicals and pesticides running off into the water table.

Scientists are also concerned that once GMO crops are released, it is impossible to retract a GMO crop from the environment. Once a crop is growing, it will naturally start spreading through cross-pollination to other fields. In this way, the GMO crop can pollute the existing agriculture system in a permanent way.

Economically, GMO farming has been shown to be more costly than conventional farming. A United Nations/World Bank study revealed that organic and sustainable methods of farming can produce 20 percent to 100 percent more food than GMO farming, because the conventional crops require less water and less pesticide and herbicide use. They also resist changes in the environment better than GMO crops. Unlike conventional crops, GMO farming also requires farmers to purchase seeds every year—since GMO seeds are patented, and farmers are not allowed to reuse the seeds for the next year. Finally, GMO seeds are often sterile and thus unable to reproduce a crop the next year.

Reducing the Health Risks of GMO Food

What should you do to avoid the health risks of GMO foods? Begin to eat organic food. If organic food is not available, then try to eat only non-GMO food. The first choice is all organic; the second choice is non-GMO. If you are eating all organic, by definition, you are eating non-GMO foods.

It is preferable to eat all organic, instead of just non-GMO, because even non-GMO food could have herbicides or pesticides sprayed on it. By eating organic, you avoid the health risks of chemicals in herbicides and pesticides.

Labeling

In the United States, there are initiatives that will require clearer labeling on food to indicate if it contains GMO ingredients. But until that effort has been fully realized, the best way to avoid GMO foods is to eat only organic food. If a food is labeled organic, it is not supposed to have any GMO ingredients.

Be careful when checking organic labels because there are different levels of organic food. You want food to be as close to 100 percent organic as possible. You could see three different labels: 100 percent organic, organic, and made with organic ingredients.

- ☐ **100 percent Organic**: All ingredients are organic.
- ☐ **Organic**: 95 percent of the ingredients are organic, and 100 percent of the ingredients are non-GMO.
- ☐ **Made with organic ingredients**: 70 percent of the ingredients are organic, and 100 percent are non-GMO.

Organic Food and Glyphosate

Experts will often point out that even organic food might have some risk of exposure to glyphosate. It could happen if herbicide spray drifts over from a neighboring field or if the previous owner of the land had used herbicides. Glyphosate can also be taken up via evaporation and come down later in rainwater. It's good to be aware of these possibilities, but don't drive yourself crazy.

There are some organizations that offer testing of crops for glyphosate content, along with certifications for glyphosate levels. One company, BioChecked, began certifying glyphosate-free crops in 2012.

Health Benefits of an Organic Diet

The Institute for Responsible Technology, founded by Jeffrey Smith, has been at the forefront of educating the public about GMOs, health, and organic foods. As he traveled the world, Smith found that people were experiencing significant improvements in their overall health and chronic health issues by switching to an organic diet—often within a short period of time.

Inspired by the stories he heard from several physicians about their patients, Smith analyzed the results of a questionnaire distributed to 3,200 subscribers of the *International Journal of Human Nutrition and Functional Medicine*. He has also reported the findings on his website at ResponsibleTechnology.org.

Focused on those who had switched to a non-GMO diet, Smith asked what type of health changes people noticed. Issues with digestion showed the most improvement. 85.2 percent of the individuals responding claimed they noticed an improvement in digestive problems when they switched to a non-GMO diet. 60.4 percent noticed less fatigue, 54.6 percent lost weight, 51.7 percent noted less brain fog (clouding of consciousness), 51.1 percent had improved moods and less anxiety, while 50.2 percent had fewer food allergies or sensitivities.

"I have seen firsthand exponential growth in allergies. And yet, when I improve the quality of my patients' diets, meaning prescribing a non-

GMO diet, prescribing organic food, their symptoms go away."
— Ashley Koff, R.D., author of *Mom Energy*

Studies on an Organic Diet

A study published in the *Journal of the American Medical Association* on the value of an organic diet was conducted in France between 2009 and 2016. The study followed the diet and health of seventy thousand people. The conclusion? An organic diet was correlated with a reduction in the incidence of cancer by 25 percent.

Another study published in the *Journal of the American Medical Association* (JAMA) found that women who ate more organic food had a higher probability of giving birth successfully when compared to the group of women who ate less organic food.

What is very encouraging about switching to an organic diet is that improvement can come amazingly fast. One study published in *Environmental Research* measured the level of pesticides in the urine of members of four families. After just six days on an organic diet, the pesticide levels in these families dropped by 60 percent. Glyphosate in particular dropped by 70 percent.

Other findings from this study included:

☐ The class of neurotoxic pesticides known as *organophosphates* dropped by 70 percent. This class of pesticides is linked to increased rates of autism and learning disabilities as well as reduced IQ in children.

☐ The pesticide clothianidin, commonly detected in commercial baby food, dropped by 83 percent. This pesticide is also associated with autism and endocrine disruption.

☐ The pesticide 2,4D, an extremely toxic ingredient (one of two ingredients in Agent Orange) dropped by 37 percent.

Studies have also shown that the nutritional content of organic food is generally superior to the nutritional content of nonorganic food. One study published in 2013 in the *Food Chemistry* found that organic soybeans had significantly more protein and zinc than conventional or

GMO soybeans. Organic soybeans also had less total saturated fat and omega-6 fatty acids.

Organic Diets Change Lives

The following experiences are drawn from two film documentaries: *Secret Ingredients* by Jeffrey Smith and Amy Hart (2018) and *Genetic Roulette: The Gamble of Our Lives* by Jeffrey Smith (2012).

Mike and Linda Gioscia have a son diagnosed with autism spectrum disorder and a daughter with asthma. In the film, they describe the changes in their children once they started an organic diet.

"We started introducing non-GMO organic food. The more we did, it seemed the better our son got. ... Over a course of months, there was improved speech and less anxiety. He kept getting better and better. Since we've gone non-GMO organic, our son no longer tests on the autism spectrum, and our daughter no longer has asthma. We look at it and say what is the big thing we changed? We changed their diet."
— Mike and Linda Gioscia, Parents

Zen Honeycutt, the founder of Moms Across America, has an eight-year-old son with autism symptoms, such as behavioral outbursts and hitting. Tested by a doctor, he was found to have high levels of fungus, which is common among children with autism. Her son also had eight times the norm of glyphosate in his urine.

As Honeycutt now reports: *We eliminated any source of glyphosate and we went all organic. Within six weeks, we tested him again and the glyphosate levels in his urine were no longer detectable. His autism symptoms were gone, and they have never come back. It's been over two years.*

Certified nutritionist Patricia Escoto describes how a change in diet helped her recover from stage 2 breast cancer—and how an organic diet also helped many of her clients undergoing cancer treatments:

"It's been eight years since my diagnosis (with breast cancer). I compete in triathlons. I feel great. I attribute the success of my recovery directly to eating an organic diet, staying away from GMO products, and eating a living foods diet that includes fresh fruit and vegetables that are 100 percent organic. That inspired me to want to bring that knowledge to other people. ... A lot of my cancer patients, once they go on a non-GMO diet, they report back to me that they are feeling stronger. They also have a higher tolerance if they are going through chemotherapy. And they're able to sleep longer, and more restful, and deeper. They are able to hold food down, and the foods they are eating are not affecting any gut issues that they might have." — Patricia Escoto, Nutritionist

While trying to resolve many chronic health issues facing her family, Kathleen DiChirara trained to become a functional nutrition practitioner. When she counted up the diseases in her family of five, she came up with twenty-one chronic diseases. She herself was suffering from debilitating chronic pain syndrome, which did not allow her to walk and made her depend on steroid injections. She also suffered from paralysis, myofascial syndrome, fibromyalgia, inflammatory bowel syndrome, food allergies, and depression.

Her son Stephen was diagnosed with autism spectrum disorder and also suffered from sensory processing disorder, digestive disorders, language disorder, selective mutism, hypersensitivity, skin conditions, and mineral deficiencies. A neurologist thought Stephen would never speak or have peer relationships. His anxiety was so severe the doctor thought he would need medication to survive in society.

Her other two sons suffered from early signs of asthma, chronic bronchitis, bloating, irritability, mood swings, rashes, eczema, and allergies. DiChirara describes what happened after she put everyone on a non-GMO organic diet.

"The quality of ingredients is really what we changed. And that's what led to resolving our health issues. We had significant changes within two to three weeks. Each symptom in each individual improved, and it happened in a noticeably short time relative to how long we suffered. Then within three months, even more resolution. And by six months, we're really looking at no chronic disease in the family. I am 100 percent confident that the removal of GMO foods, glyphosate, and pesticides was the fundamental, the foundation for why we all recovered." — Kathleen DiChirara, Nutrition Practitioner

---

The father commented on the transformation he saw in his son who suffered from autism:

If it worked that well for Stephen, from really not being able to communicate at all to where he is today, it is just remarkable. And so many more people can benefit from that if they have that information. But most of those people probably don't know that you can do that much for yourself and your children. And you really can. You don't have to rely on the outside therapies alone. You can do a lot of good, too. And it starts in the kitchen.

As DiChirara reflected on the power of changing diets, she made a few observations on why a change in diet can work:

Take away what is continually breaking down and contributing to the diseased state, and the body will heal itself. Almost everybody I talk to says, "My doctor says diet has nothing to do with my condition, has nothing to do with the symptom." And that's wrong. It's false information. I think that medical doctors should say that they don't have any experience in the area of nutrition and therefore can't comment on whether or not diet influences their particular condition. But to say that it has nothing to do with it is a flat-out lie.

The American Academy of Environmental Medicine (AAEM) is an association of physicians and health professionals founded in 1965 to "expand the knowledge of interactions between individuals and their environment, as these may be demonstrated to be reflected in their total health." In 2009, this group created an official statement outlining their position on GMO foods (https://www.aaemonline.org/gmo.php).

Because GM foods have not been rigorously tested for human consumption, and because there is ample evidence of probable harm, the AAEM asks:

- *Physicians to educate their patients, the medical community, and the public to avoid GM foods when possible and provide educational materials concerning GM foods and health risks.*

- *Physicians to consider the possible role of GM foods in the disease processes of the patients they treat and to document any changes in patient health when changing from GM food to non-GM food.*
- *Our members, the medical community, and the independent scientific community to gather case studies potentially related to GM food consumption and health effects, begin epidemiological research to investigate the role of GM foods on human health, and conduct safe methods of determining the effect of GM foods on human health.*
- *For a moratorium on GM food, implementation of immediate long-term independent safety testing, and labeling of GM foods, which is necessary for the health and safety of consumers.*

GMOs and the FDA

After reviewing the evidence about GMOs and the potential harm to your health, one question that you would naturally ask is: Why did the FDA allow GMO-based foods to have such widespread distribution in our food supply?

The answer is in the book called *Altered Genes, Twisted Truth* by Steven M. Druker. The subtitle of the book summarizes his findings: *How the Venture to Genetically Engineer Our Food Has Subverted Science, Corrupted Government, and Systematically Deceived the Public.*

Based on internal documents that were made public as part of a lawsuit filed against the FDA, the book reveals a cover-up of the dangers of GMO foods and a misrepresentation of the facts by the FDA with the purpose of rushing these foods into the marketplace.

In the opinion of Druker, "If the FDA had told the truth, followed science, and obeyed the law, GE foods would most likely never have gained commercialization anywhere."

He concluded that the development and distribution of GMO foods was done in a very unscientific manner. In fact, he makes the claim "that in no other instance have so many scientists so seriously subverted the standards they were trained to uphold, misled so many people, and imposed such magnitude of risk on both human health and the health of the environment."

Conclusion

There is enough evidence to cause anyone to be concerned about the health risk of GMO foods and pesticides in human diets. As dangerous as the risk is, the good news is that you can significantly reduce that risk by switching to an organic diet. Any buildup of pesticides that may exist in your system will quickly start diminishing when you switch to an organic diet. Many health disorders—even chronic health disorders—are found to be reduced through this single change in diet.

If you are interested in researching this topic further, or if you want to keep up with updates on GMOs, here are several vital resources:

- ☐ Institute for Responsible Technology (https://www.ResponsibleTechnology.org)
- ☐ Non-GMO Project (https://www.nongmoproject.org)
- ☐ U.S. Right to Know (https://www.usrtk.org)
- ☐ Earth Open Source (https://www.EarthOpenSource.org)
- ☐ *Altered Genes, Twisted Truth: How the Venture to Genetically Engineer Our Food Has Subverted Science, Corrupted Government, and Systematically Deceived the Public* by Steven M. Druker (https://amzn.to/3qbLtm8)
- ☐ *Genetic Roulette: The Gamble of Our Lives* film (https://geneticroulettemovie.com)
- ☐ *Secret Ingredients* film (https://secretingredientsmovie.com)

Chapter 8: Ayurveda Detox

Why do you need to detox? Due to environmental pollution, your ecosystem is not what it once was. You are inundated with toxins: in your food, water, soil, air, and even in some cookware. When you don't feel well, you will try any detox protocol you come across. In this chapter, you will learn how to eliminate harmful toxins from your mind and body to be the healthiest you've ever been.

Check out these Ayurveda detoxification methods to reduce ama (toxins) and increase ojas (the essence of pure health). Ayurveda detoxes take a multifaceted approach: diet, herbal preparations, herbal oil massages, enemas, elimination therapy, sauna sweats, red light and infrared therapy, and Panchakarma (clinical programs).

You'll also learn how to reduce or eliminate sugar, alcohol, excess carbs, fatty foods, and caffeine as well as how to detox from GMOs, parasites, and heavy metals.

Ayurveda Detox Benefits

An Ayurveda detox provides you with many benefits:

- ☐ Improve digestion and gut health (microbiome).
- ☐ Improve immunity and get sick less often.
- ☐ Improve long-term health by removing toxins that can cause imbalances and disease.
- ☐ Lose weight, or gain weight for those that need it.
- ☐ Increase happiness and improve mood.
- ☐ Reduce feelings of anger, worry, anxiety, and depression.

☐ Experience greater clarity of mind and increased focus.

☐ Boost energy and vitality.

☐ Look younger and enjoy more youthful looking skin.

☐ Get better quality of sleep and wake up easier and more refreshed.

The Ayurveda Detox

Ayurveda views each individual person as unique; therefore, detox treatments need to be customized to your individual constitution and current imbalances. The purpose of any detox program should be to eliminate the toxins that are at the root cause of disease.

Do you remember *ama*, that sticky substance that we discussed in earlier chapters that can clog and block your channels? In this detox section, you will learn how to get rid of ama; otherwise, toxins can get deposited in your fatty tissue and remain there causing chronic health issues. The accumulation of toxins is the enemy that causes disease. Detoxification methods are the friendly army that help to enliven the inner intelligence of your body and strengthen your body's natural immunity and healing ability.

If you are a beginner, start slowly. It may take a while to grasp this content. The section on heavy metal detox, for example, requires testing to be done first—and you may not be in a place mentally, emotionally, timewise, or financially to do that right away.

Decades ago, when I was introduced to Ayurveda, I took things step-by-step. When the time was right, I was able to decide with a clear mind which step I needed to take next based on my health needs at that time.

Many people have embarked on detox programs, either at home or at a clinic. Many programs are quite effective, but I often hear people report uncomfortable side effects. They might also not experience as much relief from their chronic health condition as they had hoped for.

Ayurveda works to ensure that both emotional and physical side effects are minimized. Other detox methods do not always consider the need for maintaining a balance of the doshas while detoxing. As a result, emotions can run amok. The classic example of bad detoxification is the cranky person who is dieting to lose weight or trying to go off sugar or caffeine. Other members of the household sometimes need to run for cover, so they are not in the line of fire of the cranky person's fury.

You can have minor discomfort when changing your diet or adding herbal preparations. That is especially true when you are giving up foods and vices that you love! The mere mention of the word *detox* triggers unpleasant memories for many people.

When clients say they want to start a detox program, I am thrilled I can support them. I prefer, however, that they make a few dietary and lifestyle changes first, so that they can ease into a more stringent program.

For example, if you are an all-or-nothing person, you may go from six cups of coffee a day to zero and feel great for a while—until the fatigue and headaches set in. Then you might go back to the six cups a day. One or two cups of organic coffee each day are acceptable, but more than that can cause problems for you. Some devoted coffee lovers find that they cannot drink coffee after detoxing because they notice negative side effects. More people have decided to give up coffee because it can cause severe acidity in Pitta types or create ulcers in people who are susceptible. People with anxiety or sleep issues should also consider giving up coffee.

While many detox programs ask you to give up coffee completely, the best solution is to reduce coffee slowly over several weeks by supplementing with green tea until any headaches or fatigue subside.

It is prudent to make changes slowly, even if you feel that cold turkey is best. The best approach long-term is to wean off any unsuitable substances slowly, so your body hardly notices anything is happening. This gradual change allows you to stick with a program for a longer period of time.

Knowing where you are on your health journey and where you would like to be can help you gain perspective on the commitment that lies ahead. You do not want to be disappointed if you fall short of your goals, or if you have not made your health a priority previously. You cannot change your past, so don't be critical of yourself or others. If you can say that your current lifestyle is not serving you well and you are ready to change in order to feel and look your best, then that's a fabulous starting point. Look to the bright future ahead and the value this book can bring for your life and health.

The Ayurveda Detox Program

The recommendations below should be fine for you to do on your own. However, it is always reassuring when you have support from someone who is trained specifically with these types of herbal formulas and the specific detox programs.

Dietary Detox Recommendations

Follow a three-week light diet made up of cooked mung beans, well-cooked vegetables, and a gluten-free grain. You can have cooked fruit as a snack or gluten-free, yeast-free bread. Remember the guideline of 60 percent cooked veggies, 20 percent carbohydrates, and 20 percent protein will also apply during this detox.

The purpose of a detox is to give our digestive system rest, so it doesn't need to work so hard breaking down heavy foods. While nuts and seeds are good for you, they may be a little heavy for those with weaker digestive systems.

Do not eat fried food, hot and spicy foods, cold foods or drinks, raw salads, root vegetables, red meat, dairy, alcohol, or sugar during your detox diet. Reduce the amount of coffee you drink. Substitute green tea if you need more energy. You can have a small amount of coconut palm sugar or organic cane sugar if you are used to eating a lot of sugar.

You will notice that everything listed below is fresh. You've learned how important it is not to eat anything from a can or eat frozen food so best not to cut corners unless you have no other choice.

What you can eat during your detox:

☐ Organic dried split yellow mung beans (not the whole mung beans that are green and contain the skin) and brown or green lentils, cooked. Change the beans around if you need some variety. Having yellow mung beans every day can be monotonous. That's why the other lentils were added to this list since they are lighter than other beans and easier to digest.

☐ Organic dried buckwheat, millet, quinoa, and brown or white rice, cooked. Some gluten-free carbohydrates are necessary for the body at all times, even during a detox. But only eat small amounts. Carbohydrates will give you energy and should keep you feeling full rather than hungry all the time.

☐ Fresh organic vegetables, well cooked and fork tender, except for most root vegetables. Favor leafy greens such as kale, swiss chard, spinach, bok choy, or arugula; orange vegetables for vitamin A such as carrots, acorn squash, butternut squash, or spaghetti squash; purple vegetables for riboflavin such as purple cabbage; and white veggies like cauliflower. Then, add in these vegetables: asparagus, artichokes, celery, and zucchini.

☐ Spice mixtures (*churnas*) suited to your dosha, or any spices that you know to be good for you. The key is to increase digestion without disturbing your particular dosha. Fresh ginger is excellent in everything. You can also use dried ginger, but don't use too much if you are Pitta dosha.

Detox Diet Programs: How to Proceed

Choose your experience level and follow the detox program accordingly.

Newbie Detox Program

You are a newbie if you've never done a detox before or you have an unhealthy diet. If any of the following apply to you, go with the recommendations below:

☐ You don't eat many vegetables or fresh foods. You eat mostly canned, frozen, premade, packaged, or restaurant food.

☐ Your diet is high in sugar and/or salt.

☐ You drink three or more cups of caffeine in the form of coffee, black tea, or soda. Green tea in moderation is fine. It has lower caffeine levels and many health benefits.

☐ You eat heavy foods such as cheese, fried foods, and red meats, at least a few times a week. You also eat chips, ice cream, or cookies a few times a week. You eat late at night and snack on unhealthy treats.

☐ You drink at least seven glasses of wine or other alcoholic drinks every week. One drink a day isn't necessarily bad, but its sugar and alcohol content can cause a bad reaction the next day. Alcohol causes dullness and can throw your system out of whack. Drinking alcohol is counterproductive while detoxing. So, you are better off slowly reducing your alcohol intake during your detox—or even weaning off alcohol a few weeks before detoxing.

For newbies, follow the detox diet two days a week for four weeks. It's possible you could even follow the diet every other day. On the alternate days, reduce your intake of bad foods by 25 percent. In contrast to your usual fare, this detox might seem like a deprivation diet. But the way you feel after a few days may be your turning point to better habits.

If you go to Whole Foods or Trader Joe's, you can find organic healthy treats to substitute for the treats you currently consume. Choose 100 percent organic non-GMO foods. Avoid soy, wheat, canola oil, or corn oil. For chip lovers, favor corn chips over potato chips. Limit sugar intake. Avoid chocolate bars, cookies, protein bars, and other sweets. Although too much sugar is never desired in a healthy diet, it's far worse to eat foods that contain GMOs, trans fats, pesticides, or herbicides.

While detoxing, leave some food on your plate and a little coffee in your cup. When you are hungry, opt for a piece of fruit or another healthy snack. If you work full-time, be careful. Don't try a detox while you have a lot going on at work or are under pressure. You must be vigilant in your workplace around unhealthy foods. You can't be rude and not eat a coworker's birthday cake, but you can eat just a little bit and then stop. Once you complete your detox, you can choose to have a small piece of dessert on special occasions.

That said, it's best to start your detox on a weekend to get acclimated, and then slowly build up by adding in a detox day on a workday. Otherwise, you could get grumpy at work and feel weak. Once you get used to doing a detox, you will feel more comfortable.

If you need to curb your sweet tooth, eat a few delicious red grapes that provide energy. Keep red grapes on hand, at home or at work, since they are the best raw fruit permissible during a detox. Most other fruits are too sour or cause too much gas and bloating when eaten raw. Cooked fruits such as papayas, mangoes, apples, and pears are all acceptable.

Standard Ayurveda Detox Program

If you are a newbie to detox diets but you eat pretty clean, you could follow the standard Ayurveda detox. This version is also good for the experienced detox participant, who has followed a clean-eating diet before.

This three-week program provides rest for the digestion system and allows deeper elimination of toxins. Feel free to start out one week at a time if that is more comfortable. The herbal preparations will help more when you are on a cleaner diet, but you can still take them even when your diet isn't optimal. You may cheat slightly. Just start back again without feeling bad about it.

The recommendations below should be fine for you to do on your own.

Herbal preparations for detox

You can go to MAPI (available online at https://www.mapi.com) to purchase these herbal products and find out more about them. At MAPI, you can also set up a local or virtual consultation with a Maharishi Ayurveda Consultant.

Please check with your doctor before starting any detox program, especially if you are on any medications. Your doctor should be able to help you understand if these herbal products are right for you.

Digest Tone (1 to 2 tablets before bed)

Also known as triphala, this formulation contains three powerful herbs to tone and improve digestion. Well-known in Ayurveda, it is typically taken an hour before bed, so while you sleep it can aid in toning and improving digestion. The best time to be asleep is between 10:00 p.m. and 2:00 a.m., because that is the time your body is transforming nutrients consumed throughout the day into fuel for the next day. How well you can absorb nutrients is a key to good health. It is not enough to eat healthy and high-quality organic foods if you can't absorb the nutrients.

Triphala is generally a little drying, but MAPI has added cabbage rose to help with that.

MAPI's Digest Tone can be taken every day for most people throughout their life. It is one supplement that is beneficial to take on a regular basis. Other herbal recommendations for a detox only need to be taken for a few weeks. Although Digest Tone is not a laxative and will not make you need to eliminate, it may not be suitable for people with chronic diarrhea, IBS, or other bowel issues.

To see how you respond to this supplement, start by taking one-half to one tablet before bed. Also, check with your doctor before starting any detox supplements.

Elim-Tox

Elim-Tox is an herb that assists your body in eliminating toxins while also improving your digestive flora. Toxins cannot thrive with healthy gut bacteria (a healthy microbiome). If you have a lot of Pitta dosha, use the Elim-Tox-O instead of the regular Elim-Tox.

Elim-Tox-O

This remedy is particularly good for those who suffer from stomach acidity or those who have acid reflux. Elim-Tox-O is primarily targeted toward sensitive Pitta individuals where the regular Elim-Tox may be too heating. If you get irritable or become impatient easily, go with this remedy. Negative Pitta-related emotions are a good gauge for choosing this remedy.

Genitrac

This remedy can be taken any time you have issues with urinary tract infections or other problems such as incontinence, frequent urination, or general weakness. A yearly or bi-yearly detox with this herb will strengthen the urinary tract in both men and women even if no obvious problems exist.

Guggul

If you are starting a detox program and also need to lose weight, this herb is essential. Pitta types will need to take this along with amla berry, so you do not aggravate Pitta. As mentioned before, you might get cranky or uncomfortable while dieting. Amla berry helps minimize this discomfort. Pitta-pacifying spice mixtures and teas can also help.

Herbal Teas (Optional)

If you like herbal teas and want to add an extra step to your detox recommendations, here are some suggestions:

Detox tea. 1 teaspoon each of cumin, coriander, and fennel. Steep in boiled water for ten minutes. Then strain and drink. You can keep it in a thermos and sip throughout the day. Add fresh or powdered ginger if you like.

The following teas come in tea bags available from MAPI.com. Add one tea bag per eight ounces of water.

Be Trim tea for weight loss. One to two cups per day. Follow the directions on the box to make this tea.

Raja's Cup has a nice flavor. Drink it to give you extra flavor as you are detoxing while trying to reduce your intake of coffee. It has powerful antioxidants and no caffeine.

Vata, Pitta, or Kapha tea depending upon your dosha. One to two cups per day. Follow the directions on the box to make this tea.

Hot Water Recommendation

Freshly boiled water is light and easy to digest. Sip it frequently throughout the day to cleanse your body tissues and prevent the accumulation of wastes and toxins. If you are Pitta dosha, let the boiled water cool before drinking it at room temperature. In warmer climates, let water come to room temperature, especially if you are spending time outdoors. This is great for weight loss.

Preparation time: Boil water for five to ten minutes. Use spring water or purified water.

Ayurveda recommendation: Frequent sipping of hot water helps dissolve impurities and cleanse your entire digestive and eliminative systems. The result is an improvement in assimilation of food, improved elimination, and prevention of the formation of ama.

The heat of the water allows it to be absorbed into the circulatory system and travel throughout the body. The extra warmth and fluid aids in opening circulation, dissolving accumulated impurities in body tissues, and flushing them out of the body.

People report that after just a few weeks drinking hot water, their digestion and elimination improve. They also feel lighter, fresher, and more vibrant. In addition, a significant number of individuals credit the drinking of hot water with the improvement of their overall health and the reduction of negative symptoms.

Directions: Sip hot water frequently throughout the day, as often as every half hour, if possible. The water should be hot but comfortable to sip. Even taking just a few small sips fulfills the recommendation, although you may drink as much each time as feels comfortable to you.

Heating: The water should be boiled for about ten minutes. Water that has been heated but not boiled is not considered as effective. Boiling the water allows excessive mineral deposits and impurities to precipitate out and increases the water's lightness and cleansing influence. Boiling the day's supply for ten minutes in the morning and keeping it in a glass or stainless-steel thermos for up to twelve hours is an effective, time-saving approach.

Spice Additions: A slice of fresh ginger root, a pinch of turmeric or ginger powder, or a few fennel seeds may be added to the boiling water if desired. These spices can increase the cleansing influence of the water in your physiology. Lemon may be added occasionally if it does not upset your stomach.

Abhyanga (Daily Oil Massage)

Abhyanga is the traditional name for a specific type of massage that you can do on your own (or with a professional masseuse at a spa or clinic). It is Ayurveda's most effective daily treatment to calm your mind and bring balance. In Ayurveda, any oil is calming for people who perform this self-massage. While it is best to perform abhyanga every morning, you can do it at any time of day, even for just a few days a week.

For the massage, use an Ayurvedic herbalized oil suited to your dosha type. The most detoxifying oil is sesame used in conjunction with herbal preparations. Because sesame oil is able to draw out toxins, it has inspired the phrase "open sesame." Ayurveda recommends that you massage your body in a particular direction to loosen toxins, so they move out of your body rather than stagnate. Disease begins to manifest when toxins are lodged in your tissue.

Instructions for Doing Abhyanga

1. Heat up ¼ cup or more of Ayurveda massage oil in a pot on the stove. If the oil is in a glass bottle, you can soak the bottle in the bathroom sink filled with hot water. Use massage oil best suited to your dosha.

2. Start by massaging the top of your head. However, to have the benefit of the oil on your entire body for a longer period of time, first apply oil to your entire body and then go back to your head. For all body parts, massage with the open part of your palm rather than your fingertips.

3. When massaging your head, you can be more vigorous and spend more time.

4. Then apply oil to your face and ears, being gentler in these areas.

5. Next, apply oil to the front and back of your neck and the upper part of your spine.

6. Start with your arms and use a back-and-forth motion over your long bones and a circular motion along your joints. Massage both arms, including your hands and fingers.

7. Now, apply oil to your chest and abdomen. Use a very gentle circular motion over your heart. For your abdomen, move your hands clockwise a few times in a slow, circular motion.

8. Now, massage your back and spine. Some areas may be difficult to reach.

9. Massage your legs in the same manner as your arms. Massage back-and-forth along your bones and circularly around your joints.

10. Finally, massage the soles of your feet. Use the open part of your palm and massage vigorously back and forth. Your feet and your head are the only areas where you can use more pressure and take more time to massage.

Once your massage is done, put on an old robe and slippers to do some chores around the house before showering. The longer the oil is left on, the better—twenty minutes is more than sufficient. Once in a while, when you have time, you can choose to leave the sesame oil on for a few hours. While not comfortable for everyone (since they might not like the feeling of the oil), most people get used to it.

Leaving the oil on for a long period of time is one of my favorite things to do when I don't need to leave the house. It's so deeply settling to my whole nervous system that it is a delightful experience. You will have to experiment to see what works for you. I often say it's risky for me to do an oil massage since inevitably I won't want to rush to take the oil off. Another problem arises when I jump into a hot bath; then I don't want to get out of the bathtub. If I have an appointment, I may end up being late. Of course, there could be worse problems in life.

Abhyanga should be done every day, but if you don't have time every day, do it several times a week. When detoxing, make it a priority.

If there is time, do an Epsom salt bath or some form of sweating after abhyanga. You can sit inside a steam bath or sauna for twenty minutes with your head covered with coconut oil. In Ayurveda, your head should not become too heated. Your head should rarely be inside a sauna, whether it's infrared, steam, or sauna therapy.

After abhyanga, leave the oil on your body for at least twenty minutes. After any steam bath or soak, shower well with soap and water to remove the toxins that have been coming out.

Daily Guidelines and Checklist During Detox

These guidelines should be part of your normal daily routine. However, be stricter with your routine during a detox. The exercise portion (a brisk walk) should be done before meals, not afterward. You can exercise before breakfast, lunch, or dinner—or two hours after meals.

Steps 1 to 4, approximately 90 minutes

1. Upon waking, drink six to eight ounces of warm water with lemon (Pitta types can omit the lemon).

2. Herbal preparations: Take one to two tablets of either Elim-Tox or Elim-Tox-O. If you're taking Guggul for weight loss, wait fifteen to thirty minutes between the Elim-Tox and the Guggul.

3. Ayurveda oil massage with the appropriate oil for your body type, followed by a shower or bath.

4. Yoga and meditation: ten to fifteen minutes of yoga, then meditate (twenty minutes of Transcendental Meditation if you have been trained).

Steps 5 and 6 take approximately 75 minutes, which includes eating breakfast. Add in more or less time based on your needs.

5. Breakfast:

☐ Option A. If you need to lose weight and have a weak digestion, have stewed fruit. Eat a small amount, so you start shrinking your stomach (by not eating too much at one meal).

☐ Option B: If you need to gain weight, add a few soaked almonds and walnuts to your cooked breakfast cereal.

☐ Option C: If you are medium weight and just need to lose a little or maintain your weight, you can have any breakfast—stewed fruit, cooked cereal, blanched almonds, and walnuts. But eat smaller portions than you usually eat to give your digestion system a rest.

Tip: If you don't prepare lunch and dinner before or after breakfast, it's harder to make the time later if you work a full-time job. To make meal preparation faster in the morning, you can soak the beans and chop veggies the night before.

6. Cook your lunch. Prepare *kitchari* (A one-pot meal of bean dahl, rice, and veggies, if you don't want too many dishes and extra pots). Or you can make three separate dishes: bean dahl, rice, and veggies. You can cook extra if you want to have some for dinner or a snack. Start preparing lunch at least an hour before your scheduled lunchtime, so you don't get hungry and start snacking.

If you have to go to work, make lunch before you go, put it in a glass container, and add hot water to it later to heat it up. You can also puree the food (beans, veggies, and grain together), if you have to eat during a work meeting.

If you're eating lunch by noon or 1:00 p.m., your food will not be sitting out too long or if you get to work early, you can put it in the fridge and take it out an hour before eating to let it come to room temperature. The idea is not to heat it for too long to warm it up so it can retain maximum nutritional value.

Here are two options to warm your food on the go:

☐ Elite-Gourmet.com offers a 33-ounce Warmables Lunch Box Electric Food Warmer with stainless steel pot.

☐ Hotlogic.com offers a food warmer you can plug in. Only use glass containers to warm up food, even if the plasticware says BPA free, because it may contain other harmful plastics.

Steps 7 to 12

7. Work and a walk. Work your usual hours, or plan to take some time off to rest. A short walk is fine for most people; those that need to lose weight can do a brisk walk for twenty to thirty minutes. If you feel weak, don't push yourself.

8. Lunchtime (at least thirty minutes): Wait at least three hours after breakfast, but eat between noon and 1:00 p.m. In a detox, you're cutting down on portions, so eat slowly. It shouldn't take more than thirty minutes if you are pressed for time.

9. Snack: Since you will eat less, you may find you are hungry three hours after lunch. Have a small amount of lunch or stewed fruit.

10. Yoga and meditation before dinner: ten to fifteen minutes of yoga. Then meditate (twenty minutes of Transcendental Meditation if you have been trained).

11. Dinner: (at least thirty minutes): Wait at least three hours after lunch, but try to eat at least three hours before bedtime. In a detox, you're cutting down on portions, so eat slowly. It shouldn't take more than thirty minutes if you are pressed for time.

12. Bedtime: Try to be in bed by 10:00 pm. If you have had a light dinner and you feel hungry before bed, you can have a half cup of boiled cow's or goat's milk, or almond or rice milk before bed.

Panchakarma

Panchakarma is an Ayurveda detoxification treatment that can be done in residence. Or you can stay at home and go to a nearby clinic during the day for treatment.

If there is one detoxification treatment that everyone should do, it's this one. My dream is to have clinics all over the world, where anyone, no matter their financial situation, would be able to receive these treatments. This is the real deal. Just three to ten days of these treatments is not only detoxifying, but luxurious as well. Panchakarma is pure heaven.

There are three available Maharishi Ayurveda clinics: the Raj in Fairfield, Iowa; Maharishi Ayurveda Health Centre in Bad Ems, Germany; and Maharishi Ayurveda Wellness Clinic (four sites) in India.

I've been able to do Panchakarma almost yearly for many decades. Since moving to Chicago in 2007, I still travel to Iowa once a year. Although Iowa can be thousands of miles from the lavish dwellings of top celebrities from around the country, still they travel to the Raj. They indulge in Panchakarma treatments that were once reserved only for kings and queens in India.

The cost of treatments at the Raj is extremely reasonable and the services are top-notch. Many spas try to copy what the Raj is doing and end up offering a watered-down version of Panchakarma, which can cost four to five times as much. Many guests at the Raj would attest that nothing quite compares to their services. Maharishi Ayurveda spas never compromise on quality.

Panchakarma consists of a variety of treatments that help eliminate toxins from deep within tissues. No other known treatments can eliminate *fat-soluble toxins*—toxins that typically get embedded in the fatty tissue and remain there. These fat-soluble toxins can cause disease. Most detoxification treatments that include sauna treatments to induce sweating can remove only water-soluble toxins, but Panchakarma goes much deeper and removes fat-soluble toxins.

The Raj Detox Program Removes Dangerous Environmental Toxins

Removing environmental toxins is a key way to promote better health. A scientific study on the Raj Panchakarma procedures found that fat-soluble toxicants were reduced by about 50 percent over a five-day course of treatment.

A study in *Alternative Therapies in Health and Medicine* was the first to demonstrate that a specific detoxification regimen can significantly reduce levels of lipophilic toxicants in the blood known to be associated with clinic disorders.

The results of the two-month longitudinal study showed that polychlorinated biphenyls (PCBs) and beta-hexachlorocyclohexane (beta-HCH) levels were reduced by 46 percent and 58 percent respectively after five days of treatment. Without the Panchakarma detox program, the expected drop in PCBs and beta-HCH over two months would only be a fraction of one percent. Previously, no method had been scientifically verified to reduce levels of these lipid-soluble toxicants in the human body without causing negative side effects (*Alternative Therapies in Health and Medicine*, Sept./Oct. 2002, Vol. 8, No. 5: pp. 40).

The air you breathe, the water you drink, and the food you eat are all filled with man-made chemicals and pesticides that can overload your liver and your immune system. Studies have shown that these toxins are associated with hormone disruption, immune system suppression, reproductive disorders, several types of cancer, and other disorders such as allergies.

Here are some of the treatments used in Panchakarma:

Herbalized Oil Application (abhyanga)—A comprehensive and soothing oil massage carried out in synchrony by a team of two technicians. The oil application uses herbalized oils prescribed to suit the individual needs. The treatment promotes the penetration of oil deep into the digestive tract in readiness for their removal by internal cleansing procedures.

Relaxation Treatment (shirodhara)—A soothing continuous flow of herbalized oil poured slowly and gently across the forehead; this treatment settles and balances the nervous system.

Nourishing Therapy (pindaswedena)—During this treatment, the entire body is massaged using a mixture of milk, oils, herbs, and rice. This procedure is particularly helpful to relieve pain, ease stiffness, and calm inflammation.

Luxury Oil Treatment (pizzichilli)—In this luxurious treatment, two technicians use a constant flow of warm herbalized oil to give the ultimate experience of deep relaxation. The oil penetrates deeply into the body tissues, softening and mobilizing impurities.

Stimulating Circulation Treatment (udvartana)—Using herbalized paste, this stimulating treatment helps to enliven and revitalize the skin, smooth fat deposits, and improve circulation and digestion.

Elimination Therapy (basti)—Daily gentle oil enemas eliminate impurities that have been moved into the intestinal tract as a result of other treatments. Basti removes imbalances, a vital part of cleansing.

Red-Light and Infrared Light Therapy

Light therapy, which is sweeping the market right now, is a detoxification method worth exploring. The variety of light therapy units you can purchase is mind-blowing. You have everything from facemasks that look like something out of the *Phantom of the Opera* and promise to remove wrinkles and firm up your skin, to caps you wear to prevent hair loss and dementia. If these units are the real deal, they will use the proper wavelength necessary for healing. However, they will work differently for everyone depending upon the severity of the health issue. Of course, proper diet and lifestyle will enhance the effects of light therapy.

Many spas and massage places offer treatments for full-body therapy. This full-body red-light therapy (RLT) generally consists of a box you go into from the neck down. Red-light therapy is not warm, but it has healing effects.

Infrared therapy is warm and comes in spectrums ranging from near to medium to far. These units can be used in people's homes. Other units are designed as portable saunas you can sit in, with the warmth coming from the light rather than steam (as in traditional saunas). Some light therapy saunas contain both red-light and infrared to provide additional benefits. I recommend these units which use both. Traditional dry and steam saunas release water soluble toxins, but don't provide the cellular detox that infrared therapy can.

Decades ago, hospitals actually used large red-light therapy boxes to help patients heal faster from injuries. When I broke my ankle last year, my physical therapist told me that hospitals used to be filled with them, but they got rid of them because they took up too much space. She was aware how much they helped patients and was saddened when they were tossed out. She favored them because they healed on a cellular level. Of course, it made her job easier since the patients definitely healed faster.

Red-light therapy helps the mitochondria, the power generators of your cells, to make more energy. This therapy helps cells repair themselves and become healthier, healing your skin and muscle tissue.

You can review numerous research studies at the Wiley Library online (https://www.onlinelibrary.wiley.com). These studies detail the health problems that red-light therapy can help with. Here are a few of them:

- ☐ **Dementia**: In one small study, people with dementia who received near-infrared light therapy on their heads and through their noses for twelve weeks had better memories, slept better, and were angry less often.

- ☐ **Dental pain**: In another study, people with temporomandibular dysfunction syndrome (TMD) had less pain, clicking, and jaw tenderness after red light therapy.

- ☐ **Hair loss**: A study found that people with androgenetic alopecia (a genetic disorder that causes hair loss) who used an at-home red-light therapy device for twenty-four weeks grew thicker hair. People in the study who used a fake red-light therapy device didn't get the same results.

- ☐ **Osteoarthritis**: One study found that both red-light and infrared therapy cut osteoarthritis pain by more than 50 percent.

- ☐ **Inflammation**: A small study of seven people suggests red-light therapy lessens inflammation and pain in people with Achilles tendinitis.

- ☐ **Wrinkles and other signs of skin aging and skin damage**: Research shows red-light therapy may smooth your skin and help with wrinkles. Red-light therapy also helps with acne scars, burns, and signs of ultraviolet (UV) sun damage.

- ☐ **Anti-aging**: Both red-light and infrared therapies are touted as being supreme natural anti-aging treatments.

Like Panchakarma, light therapy can detox deep into the tissues. It should not replace an annual Panchakarma detox, but it can greatly enhance one's health. Light therapy can build collagen naturally without chemicals. You can do the therapy at home. The money you save from having to pay for personal treatments makes buying a light therapy unit a good investment for you and your home.

Infrared Saunas

Infrared saunas help your body to mobilize toxins and maximize their elimination. Infrared frequencies penetrate deep into the muscles and tissues of your body. These frequencies vibrate water clusters in your body, which makes the water more mobile and better able to access body tissues. These frequencies also eliminate toxins from fat cells, muscles, tissues, and organs. This enhances cell membrane tone and functionality which, in turn, helps the cell to absorb nutrients and excrete toxins more effectively. Infrared saunas, thus, help with nutritional upload and also improve circulation.

Infrared saunas have also been shown to lower lactic acid levels, stimulate endorphins, and kill parasites, pathogens, and other microorganisms, while strengthening the immune system. Infrared saunas also detoxify cells by vibrating ionized bonds, reducing inflammation and swelling, and improving lymphatic and blood circulation. The increase in core temperature increases oxygen delivery to the cells and tissues as well as improves microcirculation and enhances immune response.

Infrared therapy makes you sweat, unlike red-light therapy, so be cautious. As I've mentioned before, Ayurveda does not recommend immersing your head in a sauna. It's best to have your head sticking out of any infrared unit. If you want to treat your face or head, use red-light therapy that doesn't heat up.

Because Kapha and Vata doshas have body temperatures that are cooler, they usually won't have issues with heat, but pure Pittas should use saunas for a shorter time, especially if they get irritable. If a sauna causes sweating, all doshas must hydrate and replace electrolytes afterwards. Coconut water is an excellent electrolyte especially for Pittas. In winter you may use Kanji water, which is the water left over after rice is cooked. Just add a pinch of salt before drinking.

Those taking medication or with any serious health issues should check with their doctor before using light therapy or saunas. Also, start with a lower temperature and a shorter time in the sauna. Build up slowly.

Benefits of Infrared and Red-Light Saunas:

- ☐ Decreases inflammation
- ☐ Increases circulation

- ☐ Relieves pain
- ☐ Relieves tension and stress
- ☐ Improves flexibility
- ☐ Burns calories
- ☐ Helps you sleep better
- ☐ Enhances immune system
- ☐ Promotes overall health and wellness
- ☐ Supports mitochondria
- ☐ Enhances energy
- ☐ Increases natural nitric oxide and redox molecule production
- ☐ Offers antiaging benefits
- ☐ Increases collagen production and reduces cellulite

The sauna I'm using right now (and recommend) is Therasage (available online at https://therasage.com). Endorsed by well-known doctors in the fields of natural health and detoxification, it offers a full spectrum, three-wave infrared heat as well as negative ions and natural jade and tourmaline gemstones. The jade in the pad and the tourmaline in the sauna generate negative ions. When paired with the full-spectrum infrared heat, the ions penetrate deep into your body.

You can buy an add-on ozone therapy device to use with the sauna. It uses healthy, safe ozone (ozone 03). Ozone therapy is an alternative approach that is an effective way to increase the oxygen in your body and concentrate it in your blood. Ozone therapy is a healing protocol, especially for anyone suffering from a chronic or acute health condition.

Enhanced oxygen treatment can quickly improve the function of your immune system, detoxify your body, and kill off harmful pathogens. It also helps hair and nails grow stronger, longer, and faster. Enriched oxygen treatments can make your skin radiate and take on a renewed healthy glow. Enhanced oxygen in your blood can give more physical energy and improve your ability to fall asleep faster and easier.

While infrared sauna therapy can have life-changing health benefits, you must still stick to a good diet and make sensible lifestyle choices. Those are still key to better health, especially if you're wanting relief from a chronic health issue. You need to implement a multi-modality approach if you want perfect health.

Heavy Metal Toxicity and Detox

To maintain optimal health, it helps to understand the environmental pollution caused by certain toxic heavy metals—and how you can protect yourself from any potential damage they might cause. As the world industrialized, more toxic materials have been used. These toxic materials have caused damage to the health of both the ecosystem and the human population.

The term *heavy metal* has been used to describe a group of toxic materials that can be very toxic to humans, even in low doses. You don't have to be alarmed, though, because there is testing you can have done as well as chelation methods that can remedy the situation.

However, it's better to know what to do to avoid heavy metals. If you are exposed to heavy metals on a regular basis, these metals can cross the blood-brain barrier and enter your brain. Such exposure can lead to the development of neurodegenerative diseases such as Parkinson's disease, Alzheimer's disease, and brain cancer.

The human physiology is most at risk from these heavy metals: mercury, arsenic, aluminum, lead, cadmium, and thallium. You can be exposed to these metals in different ways.

Mercury

Mercury can enter your physiology through foods you eat (fish, in particular), through leaching from mercury fillings in your teeth, or through vaccines you may have received as a child or an adult. The ban on mercury in tooth fillings was the first step by the medical community toward acknowledging that mercury poisoning was a health threat. Today, you probably won't find a dentist anywhere in the US using mercury fillings, while a decade or two ago, you had to specify that you didn't want them.

In fact, for those that choose to get mercury fillings removed, dentists use a special incubator, so when the mercury filling is extracted, it is instantly sucked up, so the mercury vapors don't escape into the air. My dentist even had the window open when my fillings were removed. The fillings then go into a hazardous waste bin that is properly disposed of.

My thought is simple: if you know it's hazardous waste, what's it doing in people's mouths? Today, mercury is considered by the World Health Organization (WHO) as one of the top ten chemicals of major public health concern. Why does it take so long to make that correlation?

The same with mercury in vaccines. It has taken decades to get mercury removed from just some vaccines, but not all of them. A health care professional may tell you there is no mercury in the vaccine because it goes by the name of *thimerosal*, a mercury compound. Too many childhood vaccines still contain thimerosal, as do half the flu vaccines. Now vaccine developers are adding GMOs as well.

Many parents are concerned that the scheduling of vaccines for their children are too close together, often with many given in one visit, resulting in more negative reactions. Speak with your doctor to find out what you can do to avoid negative side effects for your children.

On their website (https://www.mayoclinic.org), the Mayo Clinic explains that if a child has an allergic reaction to a vaccine, they will discontinue vaccines. But, before giving vaccines, are they testing children for all potential allergic substances? Probably not.

To be safe, research any vaccine you or your children might get. Ask tough questions. Although vaccine benefits outweigh negative side effects, it would certainly depend upon the situation, especially if your child gets seriously ill from getting a vaccine. You can request the scheduling of vaccines to be spread out, but you have to be persistent.

Arsenic

Arsenic has been found in rice that absorbed it from contaminated soil. To eliminate the arsenic, soak your rice for about ten minutes or, better yet, overnight. Then rinse the rice well before cooking. This soaking and rinsing will remove most of the arsenic. For brown rice, soak it at least as long as overnight, since brown rice tends to contain more arsenic than white rice. White basmati and jasmine rice have much lower arsenic levels. If you eat leafy greens with your meal, arsenic can detoxify out of the system more easily. You can also parboil rice so the arsenic leaches into the water. You can then throw the water out and rinse the rice a second time.

Aluminum

Aluminum can be found in food, either due to the cookware used, aluminum containers you store food in, or the aluminum cans food is packaged in. Read labels carefully and don't cook in either disposable or non-disposable aluminum cookware.

Teflon

Although Teflon or other nonstick cookware are not made of heavy metals, they have a number of harmful effects. Nonstick pots and pans are so easy to clean up, but when their surfaces get scratched, harmful metal can leach through, including aluminum, lead, and cadmium. In addition, the chemical actually in the Teflon coating is a known carcinogen. Although some brands of Teflon claim to be nontoxic, it's better to be safe and use something else.

Perfluorooctanoic acid (PFOA), also known as C8, was an ingredient in the Teflon coating that is now banned by the EPA. Chemour, the company that now owns Teflon, uses other chemicals in place of the C8 that has been banned. Even though Chemour has removed the cancerous chemical PFOA from their nonstick cookware, other chemicals used could be harmful. Because C8 in Teflon was used in other products as well, 98 percent of Americans have it in their systems. It has even been found in fetuses and breast milk. Sadly, Teflon can cause major illnesses, including kidney and testicular cancer. Even if Teflon isn't used, manufacturers fail to warn consumers that when nonstick cookware gets scratched, the underlying chemicals often consist of toxic metals or other chemicals no one should want in their system.

The best cookware to use is either high quality stainless steel or unleaded glass cookware and storage containers. Don't store food in plastic containers. And use parchment paper instead of aluminum foil to prevent foods from sticking when baking.

Can PFAS Cause Harm?

PFAS is a term that refers to a group of synthetic chemical compounds, of which PFOA is one example. The health effects of PFAS and PFOA are often debated, but a growing body of evidence has linked exposure to the following:

☐ Developmental issues, cancer, liver damage, immune system disruption, resistance to vaccines, thyroid disease, impaired fertility, and high cholesterol. PFAS have been dubbed "possibly carcinogenic" to humans by the Environmental Protection Agency and the International Agency for Cancer Research.

☐ A study funded by DuPont as part of a legal settlement with residents living near one of its Teflon facilities found that PFOA was linked to six disease outcomes: kidney cancer, testicular cancer, thyroid disease, ulcerative colitis, high cholesterol, and pregnancy-induced hypertension.

☐ Numerous studies on PFOS and PFOA on both humans and animals have shown a wide range of possible health effects, including decreased fertility among women, decreased sperm count and penis size, lowered birth weight, cancer, and—among animals studied—death.

How Can Consumers Limit Their Risks?

Exposure to PFAS comes mainly from drinking contaminated water, eating food packaged in certain materials, or using products embedded with PFAS.

☐ Avoid non-stick cookware, Gore-Tex fabrics and clothing made with pre-2000 Scotchguard, and personal care products containing polytetrafluoroethylene (PTFE) or fluorinated compounds.

☐ When in doubt, ask manufacturers if their products contain PFAS, since products are often not labeled properly.

☐ Ask your local health department if your water is contaminated above EPA-specified levels. If so, stop using the local water.

☐ Watch out for local fish advisories, and don't eat contaminated catches.

How Are PFAS Regulated?

The federal government does not currently regulate PFAS. Amid growing public concern, the EPA announced in February 2020 that it would begin the process of regulating PFOA and PFAS in the next two years (these regulations, if issued, would not apply to other PFAS chemicals). Some states with high exposure, including Washington, are pushing their own regulations and bans.

PFOS and PFOA have been largely phased out of use in the US under a 2006 voluntary agreement brokered by the EPA with eight major companies, including DuPont. However, these substances are still circulating in the US via imports.

Research on the chemicals used to replace PFOA—including GenX, which is produced by DuPont spinoff Chemours—is limited. A 2018 draft assessment by the EPA noted several animal studies showing negative effects from GenX on the kidneys, liver, and immune system.

In the EU, where PFAS use and manufacture is much lower than the US, PFOS is regulated as a persistent organic pollutant. More regulations are expected in the future.

The Bottom Line Regarding Nonstick Cookware

In research regarding nonstick cookware, as it pertains to human health and environmental contamination, the main area of concern lies with PFAS, a synthetic chemical used during the production process of PTFE coatings (such as Teflon).

- ☐ When heated to high temperatures, PTFE can start to break down and release toxic gas fumes that cause flu-like symptoms. Breathing these fumes can be hazardous to both humans and pets (especially birds).

- ☐ When cheap nonstick coatings wear out, the exposed core is typically made from a reactive metal (such as aluminum or copper) and may leach heavy metals (such as aluminum, copper, lead, or cadmium).

- ☐ Nonstick coatings can flake into your food.

- ☐ The manufacturing process for today's PTFE-based nonstick cookware involves another type of PFAS chemical called GenX, which has an unproven safety profile.

- ☐ Even if most of the industry properly handled and disposed of PFAS, it only takes a few bad apples to contaminate the environment.

Lead

Lead can be found in the water you drink (from lead pipes that carry the water); it can be absorbed through inhaling lead paint vapors; or it can be ingested, typically by children, from flakes of lead-based paint that have chipped off of the walls.

Lead is even used in makeup, particularly lipstick. If you buy your makeup in a drugstore or department store, it most likely has lead and other toxic chemicals. Some companies, however, are very reliable in providing personal care products devoid of chemicals that still do the job and work well.

The first thought that comes to mind, especially for women, is simple: Are natural personal products as effective as chemically-laden products? The answer is *yes*. In fact, products with less chemicals will often make your skin look better and more youthful since, over time, toxic substances make your skin look more wrinkled, lifeless, and dull. Even if you're not vegan, choose a vegan company when possible. Why? Because you will automatically reduce the toxicants that are found in animal products. Also, avoid soy and gluten in personal care products since they can be genetically modified and may be allergenic.

Lead is also found in leaded crystal as well as some ceramic cookware and dinnerware. Many companies, though, make unleaded crystal and ceramic ware. Search online or ask stores to research for you if they are unsure what their products consist of.

A number of years ago, lead was found in the water mains of Flint, Michigan. Lead from the city's old pipes leached into people's drinking and bathing water. As a result, alarmingly high levels of lead were found in the blood of city residents. The outcry that followed forced a change in the city's leadership, resulted in criminal charges against state and local officials, and produced a year-long effort to replace Flint's dangerous lead pipes.

The EPA asserts that no amount of lead is safe. Unfortunately, children are more vulnerable to long-term effects than adults; science has shown that even low levels of lead can impair brain development of fetuses, infants, and young children. The damage can reverberate for a lifetime, reducing IQ and physical growth as well as contributing to anemia, hearing impairment, cardiovascular disease, and behavioral problems. Lead exposure in adults has been linked to high blood pressure, heart and kidney disease, and reduced fertility.

The moral of this story: Don't trust water you drink anywhere in the world. If you live in an older house, your pipes may have lead or be corroded. And, as noted above, city water can also be loaded with lead.

Evidence-based guidance is available for managing increased lead exposure in children and reducing sources of lead in your environment, including lead in housing, soil, water, and consumer products. The good news is that reducing lead exposure has been shown to be cost-effective.

Cadmium

Cadmium can be found in food that has been grown in contaminated soil as well as in drinks, especially if you use bright-colored, glazed ceramic cups. Note: you can buy lead-free and cadmium-free cups and dinnerware that look great without the added toxic exposure.

Thallium

Thallium can be found in vegetables that have been grown in soil contaminated with this heavy metal.

Protocol for Heavy Metal Detox

Heavy metals need to be eliminated under the guidance of a health professional. If not done properly, you could get an overload in the kidneys and liver.

Panchakarma treatment and infrared saunas are excellent for moving heavy metals out of your body. Before proceeding with treatments, test your hair and blood to get a precise analysis. Then discuss your options for treatment with an experienced health care professional as well as your doctor.

Parasite Detox

A parasite is an organism that lives in or on an organism of another species (its host) and benefits by deriving nutrients at the other organism's expense. For humans, it is possible to have parasites occupying their physiologies and causing health issues.

If you don't have parasites, then you don't need to do a parasite detox. However, if you are not feeling well and don't know what's wrong, then it's worth doing a stool test with an infectious disease specialist, who can help determine if the source of your problems might be parasites. Bloating, fatigue, brain fog and loose stools are common symptoms of parasites. But it's also possible to have parasites and not have any symptoms at all, even though the parasites might be causing some damage to your health. Therefore, even if you don't have any obvious symptoms, it's probably worth testing for parasites, especially if you've recently traveled to a foreign country.

To better understand parasites, we need to understand viruses and bacteria. Viruses, bacteria, and parasites are all living organisms that are found all around us. They are in the water and the soil. They are on the surfaces of foods that we eat. They are on surfaces that we touch, such as countertops in the bathroom or kitchen, or surfaces in restaurants. The reason parasites can be harmful to our physiology is that they can proliferate very quickly, and they can cause damage to the organs of our body if they multiply into large quantities.

The first line of defense against parasites is to maintain a strong immune system and strong gut health. Following many of the suggestions in this book to strengthen the immune system and gut health will help reduce the danger of parasites.

Where Parasites Come From

Unfortunately, it seems that parasites have become more of an issue in the modern age, compared to life a few decades ago. In the past, the risk of parasites mainly came from traveling to foreign countries. In today's world, there is a risk of parasites even if you don't travel to foreign countries.

There could be parasites on food you eat in a restaurant. Typically, the risk is mainly with raw food, such as salad since the high heat of cooking should kill most parasites and their eggs. Just washing fresh vegetables and fruits will not necessarily eliminate the parasites. There are some special methods recommended to help remove parasites form raw food, but these can be tedious. One example is to soak raw vegetables in a peroxide/water solution before eating.

The problem is that even if we eat some raw food with just a few larvae (eggs) on it, those eggs can hatch and begin the growth of a family in our body. I know this is not the most pleasant topic to discuss, but it's something that you need to be aware of, in case you, or someone you know, is experiencing some health issues, and the doctors cannot figure out what the cause is. The doctors may not be testing for parasites, and sometimes the parasites might be the cause of otherwise mysterious illnesses.

Testing for Parasites

When you are testing for parasites, it's better to consult with a parasite specialist, since a general practitioner may not be able to read a stool test result with the necessary expertise. Also, it's a good idea to consult with a specialist who has some holistic health experience as well.

If you are able to start treating parasites at an early stage, you will have more success. If they have been in your system for years, then the task of getting rid of them becomes more difficult, but not impossible. Some experts claim that parasites can die off on their own after a few years, but this is not always the case.

Sometimes you will be able to see the parasites, or eggs of the parasites, in your stool. If you have round worm, you might see a stool shaped with a little curve. I have heard stories of some people noticing a worm in their stool that was as much as 12 inches long. The eggs of the parasites might look like tiny clear worms. When you start treating the parasites to kill them, you might see the "die-off" of the parasites in your stool, which means you will see shapes that are just dead pieces of the parasites, which are exiting the system.

How to Treat Parasites

First, let's discuss some food options that will help kill the parasites. If the parasites are in an early stage, you can have some benefit from certain foods, such as raw garlic, pumpkin seeds, pomegranates, beets, and carrots. These are all foods that have been used traditionally to kill parasites. Another food option is a mixture of honey and papaya seeds. This option was researched in a study, which found it cleared parasites out of the stools in 23 out of 30 subjects.

One key aspect to a parasite-killing diet would be a sugar free and gluten free diet. The parasites love sugar and wheat, and if you take away those foods, the parasites do not survive as well. Another suggestion to help eliminate the parasites is to drink plenty of water to help flush out your system.

In addition to diet suggestions, there are some natural herbs that can help.

Flora Tone: This herb is from MAPI (mapi.com). It will help support a healthy intestinal flora and contains a mixture of herbs that are known to support the colon's natural ability to remove parasites. This can be taken twice a day on an empty stomach (2-3 tablets each time).

Biocidin: This herb is from Bio-Botanical Research, Inc. (https://biocidin.com). This product helps to destroy what is called the biofilm. The biofilm is a protective film around the larvae of the parasites, and this needs to be destroyed, so that the larvae can then be killed by whatever anti-parasite formula you are taking. Otherwise, you might be killing the worms, but not the larvae, and therefore, the parasites will continue to perpetuate themselves. This herb also helps to reduce candida, which can develop as a result of worm inflammation. The recommended dosage is to start with one capsule per day and then gradually increase to one capsule three times per day.

If you are working with a parasite specialist and decide to take prescribed medications for the parasites, I would discuss with the specialist the idea of continuing to take these herbs (listed above) for a few months, along with a probiotic, so that you can strengthen your healthy gut bacteria, which have probably been weakened by the parasites.

Appendix I: Easy Ayurvedic Recipes

Healthy Meals You Can Make in 30 Minutes or Less

When I say healthy meals in thirty minutes, I don't include the cooking time since you can go and do other things while the food cooks. If you are an inexperienced cook, just dive in and don't think too much about each step. More experienced cooks will breeze through preparing these recipes.

Since I don't eat or prepare meat, I don't know how to give you suggestions on how to cook it if you want to add it to any of these recipes. However, you can use my recommended sauces for your meat and fish—and just add a few beans or legumes to up your amino acids and other nutrients essential to good health. Small amounts of legumes with other foods and spices will help you digest them well and will not cause gas. At night, though, eat fewer beans or none at all. For the main meal or snack, some beans should be fine.

Most of the meals I make are tri-doshic—that is, good for all types. However, once you know what works for you and what doesn't, adjust as needed. You will soon discover what triggers a negative reaction in you or a family member.

When I teach people how to cook, my goal is to have you become less overwhelmed preparing meals. Attitude is everything. With time, you can begin to view your kitchen as your sanctuary, a reprieve from sitting at your computer or other sedentary tasks that don't allow you to move as much as you should. Many of my clients report that cooking becomes easier with practice and that making meals is almost meditative.

Don't forget why you are spending time around the stove to prepare healthy meals rather than throw a frozen meal into the microwave—because your health and the health of your family depend upon it. You may be doing well health wise, but chronic illnesses are on the rise due to eating unhealthy foods that cause inflammation and disease. Most people wait until they get sick before getting serious about a healthier diet. Please begin now. You must commit to this lifestyle choice—and be an example for your children and grandchildren, no matter how difficult it is.

It can be rewarding to see your family and friends enjoy your healthy and delicious meals. Even if you don't like to cook, encourage family members to help you. Make it a special time to bond. You can listen to your favorite music and dance with your family during meal prep. If you make it fun, your family members will naturally gravitate to your kitchen and want to help. Even your five-year-old can contribute. Preparing meals is a great way to nurture yourself and others. When I'm planning meals during the work and school week, I keep it simple. For instance, you can have a pesto or other favorite sauce on hand to toss on veggies and other healthy dishes.

Although Ayurveda prefers food to be cooked fresh daily, you can have leftovers if meal prep won't work any other way. However, don't freeze cooked food. Try to consume leftovers within three or four days of preparing and reheat on low to preserve the nutritional value.

I dislike using frozen foods since they have less nutritional value. Buy fresh ingredients if you can. Ayurveda does not recommend precooked foods either; however, pickles, Indian chutney, and sauerkraut act as probiotics and can be used as premade foods.

Basic Bread Recipes

Grains are not the enemy, especially if they are gluten-free. Bread has a bad reputation because of the bleached, highly-processed flour that is bereft of nutrients. However, good carbohydrates are your body's main source of energy. They help fuel your brain, kidneys, heart muscles, and central nervous system. The fiber found in carbohydrates can aid in digestion, helps you feel full, and keeps cholesterol levels in check.

I recommend each meal contain about 20 percent carbohydrates. Your body can store extra carbohydrates in your muscles and liver for use when you're not getting enough carbohydrates in your diet. A carbohydrate-deficient diet may cause headaches, fatigue, nausea, constipation, weakness, difficulty concentrating, bad breath, and vitamin and mineral deficiencies.

Why go gluten-free or use spelt or einkorn instead of whole wheat? Because wheat just isn't what it once was. The purity of wheat products declined in the 20th century when manufacturers started to bleach and process wheat, which caused the gluten content to increase dramatically. They also added bromate, a preservative to hold bread together, but bromate is terrible for your health.

The hybridization of wheat also didn't help. It increased the protein parts, known as *epitopes*, that cause celiac disease. As a result, modern wheat is making people sick. Norman Borlaug, the Nobel Prize–winning wheat breeder, developed hybridization. His discovery was praised at the time due to higher-yielding wheat, but inadvertently it created a high-gluten wheat that humans had not evolved to digest.

If you have celiac disease or a wheat allergy, avoid eating wheat. Keep in mind that many foods contain wheat—such as salad dressings and prepared sauces. So read labels carefully.

Eating any grain with yeast is not good, so eat yeasted bread only a few times a month at most. It's also best to avoid baking soda and any baking powder with aluminum.

You will feel so proud when you master your bread making skills.

Homemade Bread

In most cultures, bread is served at every meal. Health and healing, however, are all about the balance of the mind-body connection. The kind of bread you ate growing up will trigger memories—and it's uplifting to your spirit to create healthy recipes from your favorite bread. I encourage you to re-create the unhealthy bread you ate into a deliciously dreamy healthy replica.

The basic bread recipe that I will share with you contains a variety of gluten-free grains. To start, buy ground flour. If you want to make excellent bread, however, get a flour grinder and a bread maker. I use a grinder, but I have not yet tried a bread maker.

I grind my grains fresh because as soon as flour hits the air, oxygen starts to reduce the nutrients. Store-bought flour often doesn't have full flavor or maximum nutritional value. Whole grain doesn't grind as finely as store-bought flour, so use the store flour for cakes and cookies for the holidays. They'll come out lighter than the grainy texture of home-ground flour.

Bread doesn't require a lot of oil (unlike cookies, muffins, or brownies where you want more oil).

Use glass loaf pans to bake your bread. Note that most metal loaf pans aren't pure stainless steel. Never use aluminum because it's bad for your health. Use ghee or coconut oil to coat the inside of the pan. Or use parchment paper so the bread is easier to cut and the pan is easier to clean.

When the bread first comes out of the oven, feel free to eat it right away. Eat it as is, or once the bread has cooled, store it in the refrigerator. Bread will last up to seven days. When you take the bread out of the refrigerator, toast it for better digestibility.

Ingredients

6 cups flour, your choice of grain
2 teaspoons tapioca powder
2 teaspoons arrowroot
1 tablespoon cassava flour (optional)
1 tablespoon chia seeds (blended with water)
1 tablespoon hazelnut flour (a binding agent)
½ cup ghee, coconut oil, or sunflower oil
a few pinches rock salt
water

Directions

Preheat the oven to 350 degrees Fahrenheit.

Use all organic and non-GMO ingredients.

Choose a grain: Millet, buckwheat, rice, oats, or coconut flour. I like more of a buckwheat flavor for pancakes, but millet is sweeter and holds together better in bread. Too much buckwheat can make the bread taste like cardboard. Use less of rice, oats, and coconut flour (see recipe details below). Quick rolled oats can also help to bind and give it a nice flavor.

Add 6 cups flour to a mixing bowl. The best mix is 4 cups millet, 1 cup buckwheat, ¼ cup coconut flour, and ¾ cup oat flour or quick rolled oats. The more oats you use, the more the batter binds together.

Combine all dry ingredients and then add ghee or oil of your choice. Add sufficient purified water to make a thick consistency. If you accidentally add too much water, add more flour to compensate.

When you stir the mix, you can either use a wooden spoon to mix by hand or you can use a mixer. Mix the ingredients until they are well mixed.

You can taste the batter to see if it has enough salt for you. It should not be a cake-like batter.

Grease a bread pan with ghee, coconut, or sunflower oil. Pour mixture into the bread pan. Do not fill to the top. The mixture should be low in the pan. It should cover ¾ of the pan. I find it cooks better that way.

Bake at 350 degrees Fahrenheit for 35 to 50 minutes. Every oven is different. When the bread starts to get brown, it's done. You can also check for doneness by sticking a toothpick into the bread. If it comes out clean, the bread is done. If it's undercooked, bake it longer.

Savory Bread

For savory bread, add 1-2 cups of olives or cooked onions, depending on your preference. You may also add poppy, sesame, sunflower, or any other seeds you like. Add the seeds to a spice grinder and grind to almost a powder or chop them up and mix into the bread. With powdered seeds, the bread will be more digestible, and you won't have to chew so much. But chopped up seeds add a wonderful crunch.

Sweet Bread

For sweet bread, add raisins and pecans. The cooking time is the same as for regular bread. If you want to make it sweeter and softer, more like a muffin, create a batter consistency between a bread and a cake batter.

Then add ½ cup to 1 cup sugar, fresh or dried fruit, and ½ cup oil and water to make the batter thinner. The thinner the batter, the softer the bread will be. But even a cake-batter consistency would not be too thin.

Muffins or Healthy Cake

If muffins are bite-size, bake for 10 to 15 minutes. If the muffins are larger, bake for around 30 minutes. If you use an 8x8 inch or 12x12 inch pan for healthy cake, bake for 30 to 45 minutes. Stick a toothpick into the muffins or cake to test if it's ready. Don't overbake, or it will come out too dry.

The reason baking is trial and error and not a science is that different climates have varying humidity levels and ovens have different heating mechanisms. Most higher quality ovens are easy to use, but still the weather and other factors often cause breads, muffins, and cakes to come out differently each time. But, as long as you don't burn it, the baked goods will generally be tasty.

Mung Bean Pancakes

High protein, digestible, and delicious, these mung bean pancakes last about three to four days in the refrigerator.

Ingredients

1 cup organic yellow split mung beans soaked overnight
a pinch rock salt
water
ghee, coconut oil, or olive oil
fenugreek, turmeric, or cumin powder (optional)

Directions

Add beans to a blender with rock salt and enough water to make a medium consistency pancake batter. The batter should be thinner rather than too thick. Blend to pancake mix consistency.

To cook, add a small amount of organic ghee, coconut oil, or olive oil to iron skillet with heat at medium low. Use a measuring cup to pour the mung bean batter into the skillet so it comes out round. Flip and cook evenly on both sides.

Add fenugreek powder, turmeric powder, cumin powder, or sautéed leeks to taste.

Healthy Snacks

What do you grab for your kids on the go? My go-to healthy snack foods for kids, big and small, would be one of the following.

Avocado on Bread

Use homemade gluten-free bread or store-bought bread or crackers.

When I travel, I always have avocados in the car, or I carry them on the plane when I fly. I bring a spoon, some salt, and a lemon. Simple Mills makes great gluten-free almond crackers that I love when I don't have time to bake bread. You can add pesto, sauerkraut, or a pickle.

If you prefer a sweeter taste, add sugarless organic jam and tahini or sunflower seed butter with avocado on bread. It's so delicious and nutritious.

Sweet Cake Snack

Bake a sweet cake or brownie (without sugar). Pack with nuts, dried fruits, zucchini, or squash.

Smoothies

Smoothies are blends of nuts, fruits, water, spices, and/or nut milks. Don't use milk or yogurt to make smoothies.

In Ayurveda, we don't use a lot of raw foods, only a little to ignite the digestive system. When your digestive system is weak or at nighttime, don't have raw smoothies. Nonetheless, some people are fans of smoothies in the morning. Ayurveda recommends simple combinations. Don't mix raw smoothies with lots of ingredients.

In the morning, most people need a grounding quality. When you start the day, if you've had some food, you will be calmer and more settled.

It's particularly important that, in the morning, you don't have raw smoothies. Drinking smoothies all day stops and starts your digestive system. It's not good for your health.

In the morning, if you want to have something quick like a shake, drink almond milk, cashew milk, or pecan milk. Or have cooked cereal or almond milk with cooked fruits.

When is the best time to drink a smoothie? If you want to have a small smoothie (no more than eight ounces), drink it at midday. But add a little oil because smoothies are aggravating to Vata dosha. Another good time to drink a smoothie is with your lunchtime meal.

Almond Milkshake

Ingredients

1 cup purified water
10 blanched almonds, soaked
2 dates or ¼ cup raisins, dried apricots, or cooked berries

If you want more sweetness, use 1 to 2 teaspoons of stevia, monk fruit, coconut palm sugar, or organic sugarcane juice.

Add spices to your liking: cinnamon, vanilla, cardamom, pumpkin spices, coriander, or nutmeg.

Directions

Soak 10 blanched almonds per 8 ounces of water. Add dates, raisins, or figs to taste (2 dates for less sweetness and 4 dates for more sweetness).

Use pitted dates or carefully remove the pits from whole dates. Some dates have two pits, so be careful. You don't want your kids eating ground pits. You could strain the shake to be sure. But usually, you will hear the pits in the blender, and you can get the bits out before the pits start breaking down.

Add cinnamon, vanilla, cardamom, pumpkin spice, or whatever you like. If the shake is too sweet, add more water and nuts. If it's not sweet enough, add more dried fruits.

Except for ripe bananas or mangoes, don't mix fresh fruits with nuts or any other foods. One exception is that you can add cooked blueberries or other berries to this shake.

Most berries, such as blueberries, raspberries, or blackberries, take about five minutes to cook on low heat. Then, let them cool down before mixing into the shake. Cooking berries on low heat is a good way to ensure that there are no parasites in your fruits. Cooked berries are also more digestible.

Here are a few fresh fruit ideas: very ripe bananas, avocado, mangoes (very ripe, cooked or uncooked).

When you add fruit, whether dried or fresh, the smoothie won't keep as long in the fridge (as compared to adding nuts or seeds). Fresh fruit seems to go sour and give off a funny taste over time. Dried fruit mixed with nuts will last longer without going sour too quickly. For optimum results, make a fruit and nut blend fresh every day.

If you want the main puree or smoothie to last longer in the fridge, make a batch without fruit and add sugarless jam or fruit before you drink the shake. A bonus: A smoothie batch without fruit can be added as a tasty sauce on vegetables or grains.

Nut/Seed/Fruit Shakes

I'm a big fan of nut/seed/fruit combo milkshakes when I don't have time to eat a proper snack or for nutrition on the go. I've recommended shakes to my doctor clients and other busy people who sometimes need to skip lunch or have a delayed lunch.

Keep a cooler in your car or at work to store your smoothies during the summer months. In the winter, a smoothie stays fine on its own in the car for a few hours.

This recipe yields about two cups of finished shake. For a pudding rather than a shake, add more nuts or flax seeds to thicken the smoothie. Keep adding water or more nuts, seeds, and fruits to get the consistency you want. If you are a chocolate lover and add cocoa you will not miss the sugar if you use fruit. It's heavenly.

Ingredients

1 cup seeds or nut combos (see Roasted Nuts below)
1 cup water
½ cup fresh cooked fruit or sugar combo

Directions

For the basic nut/seed/fruit shake, blend water, nuts or seeds, and fruit. These shakes or puddings are not an exact science. When combining ingredients, be flexible. If you use the ingredients recommended here, you'll have nutrient-dense smoothies with ingredients that blend well together.

It takes 5 minutes or less to cook fruit. Let it cool before adding it to your smoothie or pudding. Don't overcook it. Bring it to a boil and then simmer for 1 to 3 minutes, just until the fruit starts to break apart. Add a little water if you want. Then use that as part of the water for your shake.

By cooking fruit, you have a greater chance of killing any parasites. It's not only more Ayurvedic to do it this way, but you get that added benefit.

Chocolate Version: Add ½ cup or more of cocoa powder, depending on how chocolatey you want it.

Vanilla Version: Add ½ to 1 teaspoon vanilla extract.

Spicy Version: Add pumpkin spice mix, cardamon, cinnamon, ginger, anise (tastes like licorice).

Veggie Version: ¼ to ½ cup cooked veggies. Your choice of butternut, acorn, or other squashes; zucchini, kale, spinach, carrots, cauliflower, or asparagus. Smoothies make a great cover for kids or adults who hate veggies. And, if you add chocolate, it hides the green color.

If you don't like putting veggies in your shakes, no problem. If you want you or your kids to eat more vegetables, add them to a puree or baked sweet. Cook the veggies first, so they are easier to digest and make for better food combining. Add ½ cup of cooked carrots, zucchini, or leafy greens.

Berry Smoothie

Ingredients

organic berries of your choice
water
coconut nectar or sugar
cinnamon powder
cardamom powder

Directions

Cut and wash organic berries. Add the berries and some water to a pot and cook until soft. Then add the cooked berries to a blender with sweetener, cinnamon, and cardamom. Blend until smooth.

Chocolate Almond Milk

Ingredients

10 to 15 organic raw almonds, soaked
2 cups purified water
1 tablespoon cocoa powder
sugar, coconut nectar, or organic sugarcane juice to taste

Directions

Soak the almonds for 30 minutes. Then drain and remove the skin. Add 10 to 15 almonds to a blender with 2 cups of water. Blend together until smooth. Add cocoa powder and sugar to taste and blend again until everything is mixed.

This blend will last about one week when refrigerated.

Roasted Nuts

Eat a variety of nuts. You can get organic roasted pumpkin seeds or roasted cashews. Any raw seeds or nuts you buy should be soaked first and then roasted. This is particularly important for digestibility.

Below are some suggested nuts and seeds you can eat. Don't eat peanuts because they are toxic.

Nuts: blanched almonds, walnuts, pecans, pine nuts, pili nuts, Brazil nuts, macadamia nuts

Seeds: Sesame seeds, flax seeds, chia seeds, sunflower seeds, pumpkin seeds

Coconut Macaroons

Ingredients

¾ stick butter or ghee, or other oil like coconut or sunflower
1 cup flour of your choosing
3 cups unsweetened dried coconut
1 teaspoon vanilla (alcohol free is best)
dairy milk, almond milk, or other nut milk
1 cup organic evaporated sugarcane juice or coconut palm sugar

You can puree 4 to 6 dates and a ½ cup to 1 cup raisins. For less sugar, use figs and apricots. Experiment and see what you like best.

Directions

Preheat oven to 350 degrees Fahrenheit.

Mix the butter with the sugar or fruit puree and vanilla. Add flour and dried coconut. Mix well. Add a little milk until moist and small balls can be easily formed yet hold their shape.

Butter and flour a cookie sheet and place rounded tablespoons of the mix onto the sheet. Keep them rounded; don't smash. Bake in the preheated oven for about 10 minutes until slightly golden brown on the edges.

For softer, chewier macaroons, bake 10 minutes. For crispier macaroons, bake them a little longer.

If you find these macaroons too sweet, add less sugar until you get the sweetness you prefer.

Detox Menu

Whether you're doing the three-week detox from the detox section, the once-a-week detox, or you just want to eat lighter, these recipes are for you. You can puree any of this food if you have little time to eat. You could literally drink your lunch. You can cook this meal anytime. I choose this detox diet a few times a week.

Split Mung Beans

Ingredients

1 cup split mung beans
1 cup water
2 tablespoons ghee or other oil
2 to 4 tablespoons spice mixture
minced fresh ginger, leeks, garlic (optional)
fresh herbs such as parsley and cilantro

Directions

Heat a little ghee or oil in a pot until melted and warm. The ghee should not be so hot that the spices burn. Always keep heat at medium to low. When the ghee is warm enough, add spices and minced ginger or garlic and sauté briefly.

Add the split mung beans and water. Add salt and pepper to taste as well as any fresh herbs you want to use. Bring to a boil. Then cover and simmer on low heat for 10 to 15 minutes. If you want thicker beans, add less water.

Always add fresh cilantro at the end since it loses its nutrients more quickly when heated than other herbs.

Leafy Greens

Ingredients

5 cups chopped firmly packed leafy greens
4 tablespoons ghee
3 tablespoons spice mixture

Directions

Rinse leafy greens of your choice (kale, collards, swiss chard, bok choy, spinach, dandelion greens, or arugula). Coarsely chop the greens. Collard greens, kale, and bok choy need more time to cook than most other greens. If this is the only vegetable being served at the meal, make enough to allow for the shrinkage as greens cook.

Melt ghee in a large pan and add spice mixture. Sauté spices on low heat for a few minutes. Add chopped greens to the ghee and spice mixture, and sauté on medium high heat until it starts to sizzle. For kale and collards, add a little water so they don't stick, but don't add too much. When the vegetables sizzle on medium heat, reduce to low heat.

In Ayurveda, it is best to cook all foods on low heat until fork tender. If you overcook vegetables, they will be left without any nutrients and won't taste good. If undercooked, they will be too difficult to digest and may cause gas and bloating.

Quinoa, Rice, Millet, or Buckwheat with Carrots

Ingredients

1 cup quinoa
1 tablespoon ghee, coconut, olive, or sunflower oil
½ to 1 tablespoon spice mixture
½ cup finely chopped carrots or other vegetable
1 cup water (water should be about ½ to ¾ inch above the grain)
salt and pepper to taste
¼ cup pumpkin seeds or other nuts or seeds (optional)
fresh herbs such as basil, cilantro, or parsley (optional)

Only add seeds and nuts when you are not doing a strict detox.

Add fresh cilantro at the end since it loses its nutrients more quickly when heated than other herbs.

Directions

Rinse quinoa in a strainer to eliminate some of its bitterness. Drain completely.

Heat a little ghee or oil in a pot until melted and warm. Oil should not be so hot that the spices burn. Keep heat at medium to low. When the oil is warm enough, add spices and finely chopped carrots and nuts. Sauté briefly.

Add the quinoa and water. Salt and pepper to taste. Then add any fresh herbs you want to use.

Bring to a boil. Cover and simmer on low heat for 10 to 15 minutes. Red and black quinoa need more time to cook than white. The quinoa should fluff up nicely.

Fresh Herb Blend

Ingredients

These are my three favorite go-to fresh herbs, but feel free to add thyme, oregano, sage, dill, or fennel (the hair hanging from the vegetable). This gives a spectacular flavor.

2 tablespoons fresh cilantro
1 tablespoon fresh parsley
2 tablespoons fresh basil
2 to 3 tablespoons cooked leafy greens

Directions

Puree all herbs and greens with a little water. You can choose to have all your greens blended in this mixture and eat them that way. Or, if you prefer to have some greens whole, just add a portion of cooked leafy greens into the herb blend.

By blending leafy greens and fresh herbs, you release vital nutrients. If you eat the blend within 20 minutes, you can feel their power. Eating greens in this way will allow nutrients to go deeper into your cells, since cooked and blended greens are more easily digested. Ghee helps digestion because it is able to transport nutrients deeper into the cells.

Add this herb blend to any meal at any time.

You may also add sesame, pumpkin, or sunflower seeds for more nourishment. Cook them with the vegetables right from the beginning. However, seeds can be heavy. If you experience some weakness in your digestive fire, skip this step until your digestion improves.

It is optional to add the spice mixture and a little ghee to the herb blend. Freshly ground ginger can be added to any herb or spice mixture.

Winter Squash

Ingredients

winter squash (butternut, acorn, spaghetti, pumpkin, etc.)
ghee or coconut or sunflower oil
pecans
nutmeg
cinnamon
sugar or puree mix (pureed dates, figs, apricots, or raisins)

Directions

Take a winter squash of your choosing and poke a few holes in it with a knife. Place the squash on the rack in the oven or on a baking sheet. If you place it on the rack, then put a baking tray underneath to catch the drippings. Bake at 350 degrees Fahrenheit for at least 40 minutes, depending on the size of the squash. It is done when the skin becomes loose and the squash collapses and is juicy and soft.

Once cooked, cut the squash in half. Then remove any seeds and excess water. Blend the squash well in a mixer or whip it by hand with a whisk.

Spaghetti squash stays intact and looks like spaghetti, so don't mash that. You can add pesto or lemon juice and olive oil. It tastes like pasta.

Top the squash with a little freshly ground cinnamon or pecan topping. For every cup of squash, melt 1 tablespoon of ghee or butter and top with 3 tablespoons of pecans. Dry roast the chopped pecans in a pan or, for a richer flavor, sauté pecans with ghee, ¼ teaspoon nutmeg, ½ teaspoon cinnamon, and 1 teaspoon sugar (or to taste).

Apple Crisp (Or Other Fruit)

Ingredients

10 cups apples (or other fruit)
¾ cup organic evaporated sugarcane juice or coconut palm sugar
1 tablespoon flour (preferably gluten-free)

1 teaspoon ground cinnamon
½ cup water

Crumble:

1 cup oat flakes or quinoa flakes
1 cup flour (wheat, spelt, quinoa, semolina, or any of your choosing)
¾ cup sugar or fruit blend puree of your choosing
¼ cup butter, ghee, or coconut oil melted

Directions

Preheat oven to 350 degrees Fahrenheit.

Place the sliced apples in a 9x13 inch pan. Mix the sugar, flour, and cinnamon, and sprinkle over apples. Pour water evenly overall. Combine the oats, flour, sugar or fruit blend puree, and melted oil together. Crumble evenly over the apple mixture.

Bake at 350 degrees Fahrenheit for about 45 minutes depending on how cooked you like your apples. The crisp should be bubbling when it is done.

Lemon Juice

Lemon juice is especially prized in Ayurveda for its cleansing, digestive, and protective effects. It is used in place of vinegar in salads.

Pesto

Ingredients

handful basil, no stems
handful cilantro, no stems
handful parsley, no stems
1 cup walnuts or pine nuts
lemon juice
olive oil
salt
pepper
small amount water
2 cloves garlic (optional)

Directions

Add all ingredients to a blender and blend until well mixed. Pour over hot pasta. Refrigerate any pesto you don't use. You can reheat the pesto to use on more pasta.

Green Beans

Ingredients

green beans, snipped
small amount water
1 teaspoon spice mixture

Directions

Sauté beans in a pot with a little water and the spice mixture. Reduce to low heat and cover the pot. Cook for about 20 minutes.

Quinoa

Ingredients

½ cup quinoa (red, white, or black)
2 cups water
1 tablespoon ghee or coconut oil

Directions

Place quinoa in a pot. Add water and ghee or oil. Bring to a boil and then reduce to medium-low heat. Cook white quinoa for 10 to 15 minutes. Cook red or black quinoa for about 20 minutes.

Stewed Fruit

Ingredients

Use any fruit you want such as apples, pears, peaches, blackberries, raspberries, etc.

1 teaspoon coconut oil
small amount of water

½ teaspoon cinnamon
½ teaspoon ginger powder or a few slices of ginger root
½ teaspoon cardamon

Directions

Add three to four whole fruit or two cups of berries, oil, and a small amount of water in a pot. Bring to a boil. Reduce heat and simmer on low for 15 to 20 minutes. Add the spices at the end.

Detox Tea

Ingredients

1 teaspoon cumin seeds
1 teaspoon coriander seeds
1 teaspoon fennel seeds
powdered or fresh ginger
1 quart water

Directions

Bring water to a boil, add seeds, and steep for about 10 minutes. Strain and drink the tea throughout the day with fresh ginger pieces or powdered ginger.

Healthy Mexican Menu

This basic 30-minute meal plan includes pinto beans, rice, calabacitas (traditional Mexican zucchini and corn dish) along with enchiladas and tacos, which can be made on the weekend when you have more time. The inspiration for this food came when I lived in New Mexico. My former in-laws and my daughter's father, natives of New Mexico, taught me how to cook this food. I created vegetarian and vegan versions.

Pinto Beans

Ingredients

1 cup dried pinto beans
2 bay leaves

1 teaspoon oregano
1 teaspoon ground cumin
½ teaspoon turmeric
½ to 1 teaspoon rock salt
4 ripe avocados
lemon or lime
jalapeño, chopped
cayenne (optional)
shredded lettuce for garnish

Directions

All beans should be soaked overnight in water in the fridge, if possible. If not, soak the beans in the morning for a few hours. Or just proceed to cook the beans without any soaking.

If you soak the beans, the cooking time will be less, but each variety of beans is different, so check after 45 minutes. These beans will take about 60 to 90 minutes to cook if soaked and may take a few hours if you have not soaked them over night. Just keep checking on them to make sure they don't run out of water and burn. You want the beans to be fork tender.

Add hot water if the beans lose water. If water covers the beans by a few inches, they will cook faster. If you lose too much water, the beans can burn. Sometimes I prefer some juice left in my beans, but not too much.

You can also make this as a stew. About 30 minutes before the beans are ready, add 1 cup rice and some vegetables (corn, tomatoes, zucchini). Add the zucchini with about 10 minutes left so the zucchini doesn't get mushy.

Note: I add turmeric to everything, but you don't need to if you feel it will spoil the flavor of this dish.

Rice

Ingredients

1 cup rice
2 cups water
1 teaspoon ghee or olive oil
½ teaspoon rock salt

Spanish people use the short rice called *bomba*, but Mexicans use a medium rice. If you like, use brown rice, risotto, or basmati rice. Unless you are making dinner for connoisseurs of Mexican food, any rice will work.

Directions

Follow the package direction because cooking times vary depending on the kind of rice. For instance, brown rice and red rice take longer to cook.

Add rice, water, ghee, and salt in a pot. Bring to a boil, and then simmer for 10 minutes.

Calabacitas

Ingredients

2 to 4 zucchini
2 to 4 fresh corn on the cob
1 large tomato, or 2 to 3 smaller tomatoes
1 leek, or ¼ white onion bulb, chopped
2 cloves garlic chopped
red or green organic chili sauce (optional)

Directions

Cut zucchini in chunks 1 to 2 inches long until you have about 2 cups.

Manually cut the corn kernels off the corn cobs with a serrated knife.

Soak tomatoes in hot water for a minute to soften the skin so it's easier to peel. Deseed the tomatoes and remove the skin.

Sauté the chopped leeks or onions with the corn in ghee or olive oil. Cook on low heat for about 10 minutes until soft. Then add zucchini and cook for another 10 minutes. The corn and onions take longer to cook; that's why you add the zucchini last, so they don't get mushy. You want them to be fork tender, not mushy.

Calabacitas means sautéed squash, mixed with corn, other vegetables, and spices. Improvise if you want to add other vegetables. I want to be true to the traditional ingredients for those interested in that. I tend not to use tomatoes at all since I limit eating tomatoes to twice a month.

My former in-laws from New Mexico would make their own red and green chili—a time-consuming process. It's basically a ritual. They hang chilies outside their home until they are ready to prepare them.

You can easily find mild or hot chili sauce in a jar. The hot sauce is only for Vata and Kapha types in moderation—not for Pitta people. The hot sauce is not necessary for a quick meal. Most children don't like how hot these are, so buy enough sauce to satisfy the adults who must have a hot sauce. I only buy chili sauce for guests to make meals extra special, but not for a quick weekday nutritious Mexican meal.

Guacamole

Ingredients

2 avocados (serves about four people)
2 tablespoons lime juice
salt
pinch cayenne (optional)
raw garlic and onion (optional)

Directions

On a cutting board, mash the avocados with a large serving fork. Then add other ingredients and stir together.

You can have store-bought tortilla chips once or twice a month, just don't get into eating them daily. Buy chips made without canola oil that are organic and non-GMO.

Enchiladas or Tacos

Ingredients

organic corn tortillas
cheese, either real cheddar cheese or vegan nut cheese
chili sauce (optional)

Directions

Lightly sauté the corn tortillas on a hot grill.

If you are making tacos, fold the tortillas and add the beans, rice, guacamole, cheese, chili sauce, and shredded lettuce.

For enchiladas, put one tortilla flat on a pan you can put into an oven. Add the cheese as well as any chili sauce you want to use to help keep the tortilla moist. Place the pan in the oven to let the cheese melt. Add beans as a side dish along with guacamole.

If chili sauce is too hot for you, add some black bean juice when you cook the tortilla and cheese.

Italian Food

For pasta or lasagna, you can use a semolina flour pasta—the traditional pasta. If the pasta you're buying is from Italy, chances are that if you have a problem with gluten, it may not bother you as much. GMOs are banned in Europe, so eating wheat in Europe and buying products from there tends to be less of a problem. I have switched to gluten-free rice pasta made in Italy. Few people will notice that much difference between this gluten-free pasta and semolina pasta.

If you have problems eating garlic but love it, take out the thin almost invisible inner green part of each clove. An Ayurveda mentor told me that if you take that green part out, you'll have less of a negative reaction to the garlic. You can also sauté your food in the garlic and then remove the whole garlic pieces later. This will give you the flavor, but not the bad breath or upset stomach.

Although garlic is great for the heart, some Ayurveda practitioners say that onions and garlic can dull the mind. Therefore, they are rarely recommended to have on a regular basis. I believe the positive benefits of garlic outweigh this dulling effect.

Leeks don't seem to have the same effect. Since they are also a prebiotic that nourishes good gut bacteria, leeks can have many positive effects on your health. You can add larger pieces to soups, stews, and sautéed foods—and remove the pieces afterward if you react poorly to leeks.

Since individual needs vary, your diet will often be trial and error. You can place the cooked leeks, onions, or garlic on the plate after preparing food to be used by those who love them. I do that with sauces when I have guests and am not sure what they can and cannot eat.

Quick Pasta

Ingredients

8 ounces pasta (semolina, rice, lentil, etc.)
6 cups vegetables
water

Directions

You can take any pasta and cook it according to directions. Pasta is great for leftover food because it can be eaten cold. Eight ounces of pasta cooked up serves about four to six people.

Choose vegetables you enjoy and that go well with pasta and Italian sauces, such as zucchini, broccoli, cauliflower, carrots, green beans, asparagus, fennel, and spinach. When cooking them, start with the vegetables that take longer, vegetables like carrots, cauliflower, and green beans. Then 10 minutes before those vegetables are done, add broccoli, asparagus, or spinach (vegetables that take less time to cook).

Arugula is optional. People either love it or hate it. I will sometimes create an extra side dish of just cooked arugula with garlic and olive oil. It cooks up in about 10 to 15 minutes. You can add arugula to the pasta salad as well. When my daughter visits, she's always yearning for freshly cooked greens and appreciates the abundance of veggies. Some of my other guests, not so much.

Homemade Italian Pasta Sauce

Italians in Italy don't have the thick sauces laden with meat as much as we do in the US. Many regions make a simple fresh plum tomato sauce with garlic and olive oil.

One time I peeled and deseeded seventy tomatoes for a sauce to feed twelve people. Even though tomatoes are a nightshade, I can't resist indulging once or twice a month. The main thing is to have a small amount and fill your plate with 50 percent vegetables.

Ingredients

½ cup onions, diced
1 tablespoon olive oil

2 cloves garlic, peeled and chopped
tomatoes, peeled and deseeded by hand
salt and pepper to taste

Optional: peeled and deseeded tomatoes sautéed in olive oil from a jar

Directions

Sauté onions in olive oil on low heat. Add garlic and tomatoes. Sauté for about 10 minutes. Add salt and pepper to taste. Pour over pasta and serve. Add vegetables to the pasta just before serving, or use them as a side dish.

When I go to an Italian restaurant, I order primarily side dishes of veggies. Most restaurants have a large assortment of veggie side dishes on their menus such as sautéed green beans, escarole, broccoli rabe, and zucchini. Then order one pasta dish to share with the table and maybe a rice dish (risotto) without cheese.

Indian Food

Paneer (Indian Cheese)

Ingredients

1 gallon organic whole milk
juice from 4 to 5 lemons

Directions

Bring 1 gallon of whole milk to a rolling boil. Turn off the heat and immediately add fresh lemon juice until milk begins to separate. At that point, stop adding juice. You'll probably need the juice of 4 to 5 lemons.

Slowly stir to allow the cheese to separate. Let sit for 30 minutes so the cheese becomes firmer. Pour the curdled milk through a cheesecloth, making sure to catch all the liquid whey in a bowl (the whey is incredibly delicious to drink, so don't discard it). Wrap the cheesecloth firmly around the paneer and squeeze out any excess liquid.

Then run purified water through the paneer to reduce the lemony taste. Let the cheesecloth hang for about an hour as it continues to drain.

Once drained, wrap the paneer in plastic and store in the fridge, where the paneer will last up to a week.

To prepare the paneer for a meal, slice as many pieces as you would like to use and pan fry them either in a dry pan or with a little bit of oil or ghee to keep the paneer from sticking. Delicious!

Lassi

Ingredients

½ cup yogurt
1 cup water
fresh sprigs of cilantro
cumin seeds

Directions

Blend all ingredients in a blender or food processor. The mixture will turn green from the cilantro. For a sweeter taste, add sugar, rosewater, and cardamom. Refrigerate until you are ready to drink the lassi. To bring the lassi to room temperature, allow it to sit for ten minutes after taking it out of the fridge.

Spicy Ghee Sauce

Ingredients

½ cup ghee
½ teaspoon turmeric
1 teaspoon cumin
1 teaspoon dill weed

Directions

Add ghee to a pot and melt it at low heat on a stovetop. Then add turmeric, cumin, and dill weed. Heat to sizzling. Then add vegetables, rice, or lentils and stir to incorporate the sauce.

Spice Mixture

This spice mixture is fresher and better tasting than store-bought spice mixes.

Ingredients

½ cup whole fennel seeds
6 tablespoons whole coriander seeds
4 to 6 tablespoons whole cumin seeds
3 tablespoons whole fenugreek seeds
2 tablespoons turmeric

Depending on your level of digestion and heat in your body, add more or fewer cumin seeds. If you have a lot of heat and good digestion, use less cumin.

Add fenugreek seeds in the winter or for Vata or Kapha dosha as a strong flavor. People dominated by Pitta should see how their emotions respond to this heating spice. If you start to get impatient or irritable, reduce the amount of fenugreek for the sake of those around you.

Directions

Dry roast the fennel, coriander, cumin, and fenugreek seeds for 5 to 10 minutes on low heat until the seeds become pleasingly aromatic and darken a few shades. But make sure not to burn them.

After dry roasting the whole seeds, use a spice or coffee grinder to grind the spices into a fine powder. Then mix in the turmeric powder. You may also add some freshly ground cinnamon, cardamom, or pepper to taste (if you can handle the heating quality). These hotter spices might be okay to use in the winter months, but check your emotions and how your body feels as you experiment with the spices.

Ghee (Clarified Butter)

Heat one pound or more of organic unsalted butter in a pan over moderate heat until it comes to a boil. You may stir the butter until it is melted, but once it has reached a boil, do not stir butter while cooking! Cook until the ghee becomes a golden color, and the solids stick to the bottom of the pot.

When ghee is ready, skim off the white froth at the top and set that aside to eat later if you like. Sometimes you get a lot of froth; other times you don't get much. Don't eat the white solids that stick to the bottom of the pan.

Pour ghee through a cheesecloth into a clean, dry glass jar. Once the ghee is cool, set it in your cabinet for easy use. There is no need to refrigerate. Warning: If water gets in the ghee, it might turn rancid. You can tell if the ghee is rancid by the black spots that appear at the top.

Chapati (Indian Flat Bread)

Ingredients

2 cups flour
pinch of salt
water
tapioca starch or cassava (optional)
coconut yogurt (optional)

For flour, use semolina, wheat, spelt, or quinoa. For gluten-free, try millet, buckwheat, rice flour, and/or coconut flour. Coconut yogurt may help the consistency for gluten-free grains.

Directions

Semolina, spelt, or wheat will produce the softest and best-tasting chapatis. Spelt and quinoa as well as the gluten-free mix of millet, buckwheat, and oats, produce a rougher texture. Add cassava or tapioca starch to smooth this texture. Add a pinch of salt to the flour. Then add enough water to make dough that is moist and sticky.

Baste the dough with oil and wrap it in plastic. Let the dough sit in a warm area for an hour. This helps the dough roll out better.

After the dough rests, tear off egg-size pieces of dough and roll out each piece flat on a very dry floured surface. The dough doesn't have to look beautifully round. It will taste good no matter what the shape. For fun, let your kids help you roll the dough out.

Preheat a pan. A good old-fashioned iron pan works best. Make sure the pan is pure iron and not made with mixed metals that can be bad for your health. Never use nonstick ware.

Put the rolled-out dough on a heated pan. After a few minutes, flip the chapati and cook the other side. Since pans differ greatly, you'll have to practice making a perfect chapati. If it comes out too hard, dip it in soup, since it will be more like a cracker than a chapati. If you under cook it, put the chapati over a flame and leave it there briefly. On a good day, the chapati will puff up. When that happens, it usually tastes great. Eat it with a drizzle of extra virgin olive oil or ghee.

Incompatible Foods

This list of foods offers tremendous wisdom. If you can follow these guidelines most of the time, it will benefit you greatly. Once in a while you can indulge in combining incompatible foods, but stick with compatible foods most of the time.

When eating the bold foods in the list below, avoid eating incompatible foods for at least an hour afterwards. Eating incompatible foods causes various types of ama, which are impurities caused by improperly digested foods. Accumulation of ama acts as the seed for most diseases, including allergies, chronic skin problems, and high cholesterol.

Eggs—Do not eat with milk, yogurt, melons, cheese, fruits, potatoes, tomatoes, or eggplant.

Honey—Do not eat with ghee in equal portions.

Nightshades (potatoes, tomatoes, eggplant)—Do not eat with yogurt, milk, melons, or cucumbers.

Raw Fruit—All raw fruit should be eaten separately. You can have a meal about a half an hour after eating a piece of raw fruit. However, do not combine raw fruit with starches, meats, and legumes. Today, smoothies are our modern-day healthy go-to drink, but a lot of bad food combining happens when creating most smoothies. Check out the Ayurveda smoothie recipes earlier in this appendix for better combinations.

Yogurt—Do not eat with milk, sour fruits, melons, fish, starches, cheese, or bananas. The only exception is mango, which is the only fruit that can be eaten with milk or yogurt.

Milk

Milk causes the most problems with other foods. Many lactose intolerances are actually due to poor quality milk (highly processed) or to poor food combining.

It's best to drink warm milk by itself an hour or more before or after other foods.

If you drink milk within 45 minutes of milking it from the cow, you don't have to boil it. This is milk at its best: easily digestible and nutritious.

Drinking cold milk right from the refrigerator is an allergic reaction waiting to happen, especially if the milk contains GMOs or has been pasteurized and homogenized.

If you eat milk with foods that are incompatible and the milk is not raw and organic, it's double trouble for sure.

Do not eat with green leafy vegetables (spinach, kale, broccoli, arugula).

Do not eat with alcohol, fermented foods of any kind (soy sauce, balsamic vinegar, apple cider vinegar, or salad dressings made with vinegars), fermented herbal supplements (including tinctures, especially with alcohol), citrus foods (oranges, grapefruit, pineapple, lemons), and pickled foods (Indian chutneys, pickles, sauerkraut).

Do not eat with eggs or with baked goods containing eggs (breads, cakes, cookies). Baked goods without eggs are fine.

Do not eat with meat (beef, chicken, pork, turkey, fish). Some cream is okay because it's fat like butter.

No raw fruits can be eaten with milk except mango. Jams and cooked fruits in pies are fine.

Do not eat milk with foods containing salt.

Do not eat with fish or with sea vegetables such as seaweed.

Do not combine milk and yogurt.

Appendix II: Recommendations for Common Health Issues

This book has been offering health tips to improve your health, so the recommendations for the following health issues will be short and concise.

For general health guidelines refer to my eight pillars for perfect health described in chapters one through eight. Follow the guidelines for your body type and add these specific recommendations based on your current health issues. You can combine recommendations when needed. Also, note that some recommendations can apply to more than one health issue.

Anxiety

Eat meals in a timely manner, especially breakfast (don't skip it). You may need two small snacks in-between meals, but don't overeat. If you are overweight and need to lose weight, be careful. Some people don't eat enough when they are anxious and, thus, become thin while others eat too much and gain weight. There needs to be a balance.

Take two tablets twice a day of Worry-Free Herbal Tablets after breakfast and lunch.

Drink Vata herbal tea. However, in the summer or in warmer climates, drink Pitta herbal tea. They are both very calming.

Avoid raw and cold food except sweet ripe fruits in the summer. Cooked or stewed fruit is fine. Eat healthy foods. Because squash is grounding, eat butternut, acorn, and any other squashes. Also, eat leafy greens and a variety of vegetables with powerful antioxidants.

Eat nuts and seeds that appeal to you, except at night. Blanched almonds and walnuts are the best, but you can also eat Brazil nuts, cashews, pistachios, and other nuts and seeds. However, if you have lots of Kapha in your constitution and need to lose weight, stick with just blanched almonds and walnuts. Kapha types can handle seeds better than heavy nuts, especially pumpkin seeds. Sesame and sunflower seeds are also good for grounding. Small amounts of these seeds at breakfast and lunch or for a snack are fine.

Massage daily with oil, or at least a few times a week. Put oil on your head and the soles of your feet before bed. You can do oil massage during the day if you don't need to go anywhere or if you Zoom for work meetings. Oil massage is very calming to the nervous system.

Arthritis

Arthritis is a common health issue, primarily caused by inflammation (in Ayurveda terms, ama) in the joints. One needs to reduce inflammation or ama in the joints through diet and herbal preparations.

For a specific diet to help with arthritis, follow the overall guidelines in this book for an Ama-reducing diet.

Some wonderful herbal preparations to lend support are:

Flexcel – Bone and Joint Management: From MAPI.com. Arthritis sufferers have found reduced pain, inflammation, and stiffness from this herb.

Joint Soothe II: From MAPI.com. A therapeutic massage oil to place on the areas where there is pain.

Digest Tone: From MAPI.com. This helps keep the digestion in check, which can reduce Ama in the system.

Colds

The common cold is just that: very common, especially during the cold and flu season in the winter. If you start to get the sniffles and a runny nose, the faster you act, the more you can reduce the risk of the cold getting worse.

Get plenty of sleep and rest.

Drink lots of fluids. Don't drink cold liquids. Drink warm teas, even in the summer. Drink green tea if you must work but require more energy.

Drink Sniffle Free herbal tea (available from MAPI.com). Add extra dried ginger powder or fresh ginger to the tea, especially if you have a strong cough with your cold.

Stop eating sugar, fried foods, dairy, and heavy foods immediately when you feel a cold coming on.

Create a spice mix. Combine one teaspoon each of ginger, turmeric, cinnamon, cardamom, and cloves. After mixing, store the spice mix in a glass jar with an airtight lid. Take one teaspoon of the mix with a little honey and warm water. Do not use hot water. If you don't add honey, put the mix on your tongue and swallow with warm water. Or you can add the mix to hot water without honey and drink it.

Constipation

Add fiber. Include more fiber in your diet from fruits and vegetables.

Increase fluids. Drink more water and warmer fluids throughout the day.

Reduce stress. Practice Transcendental Meditation to reduce stress.

Digest Tone. From MAPI.com. Supports healthy elimination. Take two tablets one hour before bed.

Depression

Check your B12 and D3 levels and supplement as needed. Take extra zinc and other B-vitamins.

Take a good probiotic. Eat one teaspoon of sauerkraut and a small pickle slice that has not been cured in vinegar with your lunch meal.

Avoid fried and heavy foods. Avoid sugar completely. Instead, use Stevia, monk fruit, and cinnamon to sweeten teas and desserts.

Use stimulating spices such as black pepper, ginger, and cumin.

Take two Blissful Joy Herbal Tablets twice a day after breakfast and dinner (available from MAPI.com).

Walk briskly in the sun in the early morning. Even winter sun is helpful. If you cannot walk in the sun, do other aerobic exercises for twenty to thirty minutes a day.

Massage with Garshan Gloves (gloves made of raw silk). Massaging with these gloves stimulates digestion and improves energy and mood.

Don't overeat. Eat three balanced meals. If hungry, you can eat light fruit snacks in between meals.

Stay in touch with friends who are uplifting and supportive. Join clubs where you can engage with people. Being alone and isolated is not helpful when you are depressed. You will feel better if you engage with other people or get out and have some fun.

Diarrhea

Diarrhea can be caused by a variety of things. Some common causes are: many over the counter and prescription medications, poor diet, lifestyle, and stress. Diarrhea can be difficult to treat for many people.

Reduce Stress. If stress is a main cause, then practicing the Transcendental Meditation technique would be a strong recommendation.

Daily Probiotic. Another general recommendation, which I have found to be helpful in some cases, is to take a good probiotic. I have had good experiences with clients, who have tried a probiotic called GutHealth Digestion & Microbiome Support from Arbonne, which includes ginger in its formulation, which helps to settle the stomach down. One lady found this probiotic significantly improved her case of severe diarrhea.

Pitta pacifying diet. Follow a pitta pacifying diet, as described earlier in this book.

Check for parasites. Check with a doctor for bacteria or parasites.

Fever

Feed a cold and starve a fever is exactly what Ayurveda would say. When a fever appears, get plenty of rest and drink a lot of fluids, but it's probably better to fast. A fever is the body's way of telling you it's fighting an infection.

Get plenty of rest.

Drink lots of liquid.

Fast, if you can. Or eat less food.

Enjoy a cool bath.

Massage your body with coconut oil, which is cooling. It may make you feel better.

If the fever gets dangerously high, go to the emergency room (ER) right away. Most people find that as soon as a fever peaks, it can drop very quickly. Other times, a fever can take three to four days to come back to normal.

Fibromyalgia

Fibromyalgia is a Vata imbalance, primarily related to stress. The body is unable to recover quickly from stress, so toxins build up in people's nerves. You can follow many of the recommendations for depression to minimize stress and inflammation.

High Blood Pressure

Take BP Tablets from MAPI.com.

Do TM. Practice the Transcendental Meditation technique, which is known to relieve stress.

Exercise. Both yoga and regular exercise help to relieve stress.

Reduce work-related stress, as well as family stress.

Cut salt intake. Also eat less red meat and cheese.

High Cholesterol

Many people who eat a healthy diet could still have high cholesterol because sometimes high cholesterol is stress-related. So, diet and lifestyle are crucial.

Do TM. Practice the Transcendental Meditation technique, which is known to reduce cholesterol with regular practice.

Avoid trans fats. Use ghee instead of butter, in moderation. Olive oil is also a good oil to use for salads. But don't cook with olive oil using high heat. Avoid butter, fried foods, hard cheeses, and red meat. A small amount of fresh cheese at lunch is fine.

Don't overwork yourself.

Exercise. Take time for aerobic exercises, fast walking, biking, dancing, or other activities you like to do.

Supplement with Cholesterol Protection (available from MAPI.com).

Irritable Bowel Syndrome (IBS)

IBS can include both diarrhea and constipation. For suggestions on treating IBS, diarrhea, and constipation, see the sections on Diarrhea and on Constipation.

Migraine Headaches

There can be many reasons you experience head pressure or headaches. Headaches are mostly related to stress, diet, and lifestyle. I typically see headaches in people under pressure at work. They are often overworked and soon develop sleep issues. Due to lack of sleep, they increase their caffeine use and overstimulate, which makes their sleep worse. Many women get migraines due to hormonal changes that get exacerbated during stressful situations.

The International Headache Society defines chronic migraine as experiencing more than fifteen headache days per month over a three-month period, with more than eight headaches being migraines. Episodic migraine is a migraine subtype, defined as less than fifteen headache days per month. From an Ayurveda perspective consider diet and lifestyle changes as more serious health issues can develop with chronic migraines.

Those with migraines or any type of headache, frequent or occasional, will benefit from the recommendations below.

For the Kapha-related sinus headache, refer to the sinus section below. Sinus headaches are at the front of the forehead; Pitta headaches are tension headaches at the temples; and Vata headaches are at the back of the head. If you experience pressure in all three areas, rest and follow the guidelines for all three types of headaches. Also take a day or more off from work.

When a dosha is out of balance due to stress, headaches can arise.

Vata Type Headache (having pressure in the back of the head)

Nasya: Putting herbalized oils in your nose is the best way to settle your mind and ease most headaches. Use Clear and Soothe nose oil (available from MAPI.com). Take a few drops and massage it into your nostrils with your clean pinky finger. Do this fifteen minutes before a meal or two hours after a meal. Don't take a shower right after using nose oil.

Oil massage with Vata Massage Oil (from MAPI.com). Warm up ¼ cup of oil. If it is summer and you feel overheated, you can use Pitta Massage Oil. Do an oil massage by applying the oil to the entire body first so it can stay on as long as possible. You can even apply the oil to your hair and scalp and sleep with the oil on your head and feet. It's very calming.

Yoga and exercise reduce stress and can often ease headaches as well.

Go to bed by 10:00 p.m. Strive for at least seven to eight hours of sleep.

Sinus Problems

Avoid dairy, fried foods and excess sugar. If you are not lactose intolerant, you can take small amounts of ghee (clarified butter) at breakfast or lunch and fresh cheese at lunch only. But it's better to avoid all dairy when sinus issues are acute. Ease in with dairy when sinus problems clear up.

Nasya: Use a nose oil two to three times a day. You can switch between MP 16 and Clear and Soothe oils from MAPI.com. Take a few drops and massage it into your nostrils with your clean pinky finger. Do this fifteen minutes before a meal or two hours after a meal. Don't take a shower right after using nose oil.

Take Sinus Protection Plus Herbal Tablets available at MAPI.com. If you need something stronger, take two MA 290 tablets twice a day (also available from MAPI.com).

Use a saline solution only once a week, at least a few hours before or after using nose oil. Don't use them together.

Make sure your digestion is good. Don't eat late at night or graze throughout the day. Inappropriate eating can disrupt digestion and cause sinuses to worsen.

Drink ginger tea. You can also drink Vata, Pitta or Kapha teas based on your dosha quiz. Sniffle Free tea is also excellent (available from MAPI.com).

Do a steam inhalation by adding a few drops of Clear Breathe (available from MAPI.com) to a large pot of hot water. Put a towel over your head and take deep breaths through your nose. The water should not be so hot that it burns your face, and also check to see that the drops are not too strong for you. If it's your first time, don't put your face too deep into the steam. The drops can be strong for some people and so ease into it slowly. You can blow your nose or take a break in between inhaling the steam. You will feel great afterwards.

Thyroid Issues

Thyroid issues, which are common, can disrupt the endocrine system. Here are some factors that may contribute to the problem:

Drinking water that is not purified. The cheapest way to get decent water is to use a Reverse Osmosis (RO) system that hooks up right to your sink. Call American Choice Water in Fairfield, Iowa, at 641-472-7823. Besides offering the most reasonably priced units, they can hook up a unit under the sink with the help of a plumber. Or they can show you how to do it. Their systems also add minerals back into the water, so you don't have to buy mineral replacements or mineral water.

Get a Natural Shower Filter (available from NaturallyFiltered.com) that you can switch out for your shower head. Such filters can protect you from toxins in local water supplies.

Hypothyroidism

Hypothyroidism, also called underactive thyroid disease, can lead to an autoimmune disorder called Hashimoto's disease. Here are a few things you can do to protect yourself from thyroid problems:

Eat a gluten-free diet. And eat more fresh foods and lots of vegetables.

Add iodine to your diet. Since so many people now use sea salt or rock salt that doesn't contain iodine, it pays to supplement with iodine. As little as one drop per day of liquid iodine is sufficient. You don't need more than that. Look for a bottle labeled 150 mcg, Iodine.

Use Thyroid Support (available from GaiaHerbs.com). The capsules combine ashwagandha, seaweed, kelp, and Schisandra. Adults should take two capsules in the morning and one capsule in the evening, between meals.

Take an Ayurveda herb. To supplement with this herb, you first need to consult a Maharishi Ayurveda wellness consultant. If you have a serious thyroid problem, take both Thyroid Support and the Ayurveda herb.

Reduce stress. Get plenty of rest and aerobic exercise.

Hyperthyroidism

Hyperthyroidism, also called overactive thyroid disease, can lead to Grave's disease. If your thyroid is overactive, you have too much iodine, so you need to reduce it.

Avoid salt, except sea salt or rock salt in small amounts (as long as they don't contain iodine).

Eat less often in restaurants, where food is often oversalted.

Avoid foods with iodine, which can be found in less obvious places, such as cough syrups, some medicines, vitamins, seaweed, and seaweed-based supplements. Check labels carefully to ensure iodine isn't an ingredient.

Index

About the Author

Laurina Carroll has been practicing the Transcendental Meditation technique since 1986 and has been teaching it since 1997. In December 2007, she moved to the Chicago area after she married her husband Bolton Carroll.

Previously, Laurina lived in Germany teaching Transcendental Meditation and working as a Maharishi Ayurvedic Wellness Consultant in one of the most reputable Maharishi Ayurvedic clinics in Europe. During this time, her passion for Maharishi Ayurvedic Medicine grew strong so she moved back to the U.S. for further training.

Laurina earned a B.A. in Maharishi Ayurvedic Medicine and a Masters in Maharishi Vedic Science from Maharishi University of Management in Fairfield, Iowa. She also worked at the Raj Health Spa as a lecturer and health coach.

Laurina continues to lecture as well as offer wellness seminars and webinars. Laurina also provides Nutrition & Lifestyle Consultations that include individualized recommendations for Ayurvedic diet, herbal products, yoga exercises, plus daily and seasonal routines that support good health.